STRESS AND ITS RELATIONSHIP
TO HEALTH AND ILLNESS

BEHAVIORAL SCIENCES
FOR HEALTH CARE PROFESSIONALS

Michael A. Counte, Series Editor

During the 1970s there was a rapid growth in the amount of behavioral science instruction included in the training of physicians, nurses, dentists, pharmacists, and other health care professionals. New faculty members were put on staffs at medical centers, curricula were devised, and on occasion, new departments were created to support a diverse group of behavioral scientists.

The new emphasis on behavioral science in the education of health care professionals and the inclusion of a behavioral science section in certification examinations have generated a need for clinically relevant text materials. This series responds to that need by providing general, yet concise, introductions to common topical areas in behavioral science curricula, linking concepts and theories to clinical practice.

The authors of the series volumes are behavioral scientists with considerable experience in the education of health care professionals. Most of them are also clinicians, and their varied experience enables them to present their topics in a readable fashion. The content of the texts presumes only a very basic knowledge of the behavioral sciences, and emphasis is placed on the practical implications of research findings for health care delivery.

It is our hope that this multivolume approach will allow each instructor to select the books most pertinent to his or her particular curriculum. The division of topics was planned to enhance the overall flexibility of the information being presented.

Titles in This Series

Also of Interest

†Available in hardcover and paperback.

STRESS AND ITS RELATIONSHIP
TO HEALTH AND ILLNESS

Linas A. Bieliauskas, Ph.D.
Rush–Presbyterian–St. Luke's Medical Center

What is the relationship between stress and illness? How does stress affect immune responsivity? Why do some people cope better than others? Questions like these have generated considerable research during the last forty-five years. In this book, Dr. Linas A. Bieliauskas reviews the most significant stress-illness research and traces the evolution of stress theory, emphasizing such areas as hormonal responses to stress and the cognitive and social factors that affect people's abilities to cope successfully with stressful situations, including illness.

In addition to examining how each individual's history relates to his or her reactions to life events, Dr. Bieliauskas takes a closer look at some specific psychophysiological reactions to stress—headaches, back pain, asthma, ulcers, and heart disease. He also discusses stress-related diseases such as cancer, rheumatoid arthritis, Grave's disease, psychological disturbances, and immune-related illnesses. The book concludes with a discussion of how the findings of stress-illness research can be applied in the clinical setting. An extensive bibliography has been included to encourage further exploration of the topics discussed.

Dr. Linas A. Bieliauskas is director of clinical training and assistant professor of psychology at Rush–Presbyterian–St. Luke's Medical Center in Chicago.

BEHAVIORAL SCIENCES FOR HEALTH CARE PROFESSIONALS

STRESS AND ITS RELATIONSHIP TO HEALTH AND ILLNESS

Linas A. Bieliauskas, Ph.D.

Rush–Presbyterian–St. Luke's Medical Center

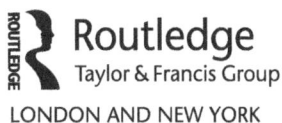

Routledge
Taylor & Francis Group

LONDON AND NEW YORK

First published 1982 by Westview Press, Inc.

Published 2019 by Routledge
52 Vanderbilt Avenue, New York, NY 10017
2 Park Square, Milton Park, Abingdon, Oxon OX14 4RN

Routledge is an imprint of the Taylor & Francis Group, an informa business

Library of Congress Cataloging in Publication Data
Bieliauskas, Linas A.
  Stress and its relationship to health and illness.
  (Behavioral sciences for health care professionals)
  Bibliography: p.
  Includes index.
  1. Medicine, Psychosomatic.   2. Stress (Physiology)   3. Stress (Psychology)
I. Title.   II. Series.
RC49.B48   616.07'1   81-14809
                                        AACR2

ISBN 13: 978-0-367-28898-3 (hbk)
ISBN 13: 978-0-367-30444-7 (pbk)

To the most important stress mediators in my life,
my wife, Britt, and my children

CONTENTS

TABLES AND FIGURES

Tables

Figures

STRESS AND ITS RELATIONSHIP
TO HEALTH AND ILLNESS

1

INTRODUCTION TO THE
CONCEPT OF STRESS

BACKGROUND AND DEFINITION OF STRESS

To discuss the relationship between stress and health status, it is first necessary to define the term "stress." This is not a mundane issue, because the term "stress" is popularly used to refer to a wide range of physiological changes, psychological states, and environmental pressures in the health/illness literature. Stress was first described as a biological syndrome by Selye (1936, p. 32):

> Experiments on rats show that if the organism is severely damaged by acute non-specific nocuous agents such as exposure to cold, surgical injury, production of spinal shock . . . a typical syndrome appears, the symptoms of which are independent of the nature of the damaging agent . . . and represent rather a response to damage as such.

This syndrome is the manifestation of a state called "stress" that included all the specific changes induced within the biological system of an organism. That which produces this state of stress is called the "stressor." The primary emphasis of Selye's observation was that stress shows itself as a measurable organismic reaction although it may be "unspecifically induced"; that is, it is a general reaction that occurs in response to any number of different stimuli (Selye, 1956). The biological reaction to which Selye referred was characterized by a general increase in the production of certain hormones from the pituitary and adrenal glands that augmented or ameliorated the mobilization of bodily defenses against different stressors (Selye, 1971). We will discuss the biological characteristics of this reaction more specifically in the next chapter.

Selye saw the stress reaction as an adaptive syndrome of the organism in response to external stressors. The form this syndrome takes is known as the General Adaptation Syndrome (GAS) and is depicted in Figure 1. The GAS consists of three phases. Upon confrontation with a stressor, the organism enters the first phase, the *alarm reaction,* in which overall resistance to a stressor initially decreases, although bodily defenses—for example, inflammation—are mobilized. If the

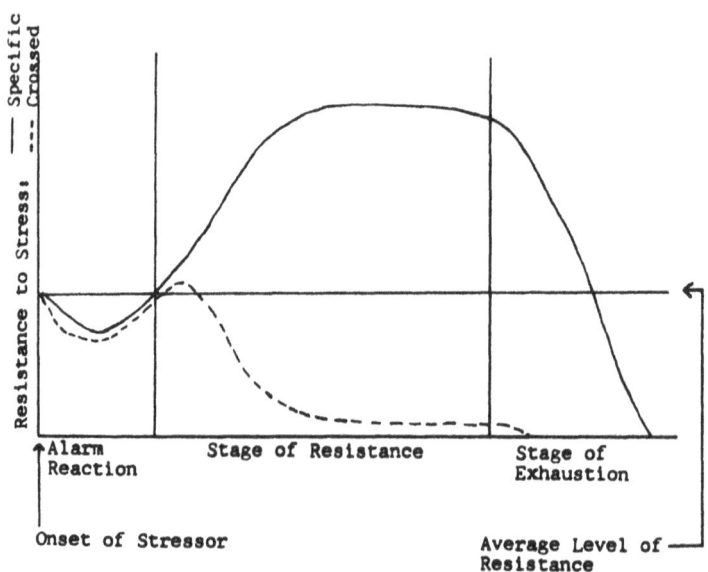

FIGURE 1. The General Adaptation Syndrome. (After Selye, 1946. Reproduced by permission of The Endocrine Society.)

stressor is very intense at this point or if many additional stressors are present, resistance diminishes to zero and the organism ceases to function. During the second phase, the *stage of resistance,* the organism adapts to the presence of the stressor and maintains itself. The stressor can even increase in magnitude during this stage without causing obvious harm. Bodily defenses are effective, and the organism either main-tains these defenses or tolerates the presence of the stressor without extended use of direct defenses. For example, a fever is a direct defensive inflammatory response to a viral pathogen. However, if maintained over extended periods, it might itself harm the organism. Therefore, a pathogen might be tolerated by the body without a direct defensive reaction, as in the case of viral infections that continue over time without any evidence of fever. In such cases, the organism is resisting the pathogen passively by tolerating it rather than actively by fighting it. Nevertheless, whether the organism resists a stressor actively or passively, its capacity to do so is finite; the presence of a stressor over an extended period will deplete the organism's resistance capacity and eventually lead to breakdown or death during the third phase, the *stage of exhaustion.* Of course, the GAS is a conceptual description of the typical reaction to a stressor and is not intended as a specific depiction of exact organismic symptoms and biological changes.

While the GAS is intended to buttress an organism's resistance to a particular stressor, it also necessarily alters the physiological balance that prevailed before the stressor appeared. This bodily change may have direct deleterious consequences for the organism if the GAS is maintained over extended periods. Selye (1956) described these negative conse-quences as "diseases of adaptation," although he admits the term is less than precise. In addition, the GAS may either in-crease or decrease potential resistance to another stressor, depending on the circumstances (Selye, 1946).

As mentioned above, an organism can respond to the presence of a stressor by direct defense or by tolerance. This dual action of the stress response is theorized to result in *crossed resistance* or *crossed sensitization* to additional stressors (Selye, 1952). Initially, exposure to a systemic stressor increases resistance to that stressor and provides an already mobilized capacity to cope with other stressors of a similar nature (crossed resistance). However, this exposure to a systemic stressor may also lead to the development of a tolerance to stressors and thus a diminished capacity to deal with additional stressors of a different nature (crossed sensitization). For example, if a tolerance is developed for the presence of a particular viral pathogen, the organism might not be able to combat an ensuing invasion of a bacterial pathogen (see Figure 1).

This traditional conceptualization of stress, then, views it as a specific biological syndrome that is a response to nonspecific damaging agents (stressors). The response has a particular timeframe (the GAS), and its activation by one stressor may have implications for the organism's capacity to resist other stressors (crossed resistance or crossed sensitization). This view of stress is still widely accepted, but there is evidence that it is oversimplified.

The idea that stress is a purely biological response has been challenged by Mason (1971), who asserted that a single biological response to a wide variety of stimuli is difficult to explain on a physiological basis. In a series of experiments, he demonstrated that the general stress response was dependent on psychological parameters surrounding the stressors. By controlling the degree of discomfort, the pleasantness, or sudden versus gradual appearance of stressors, Mason was able to show that such factors could account for the presence or absence of the biological stress response even if the actual stressors—say, workload or lack of nutrition—remained unchanged. Thus, Mason felt that "the stress concept should not be regarded primarily as a physiological concept but rather as a behavioral one" (1971, p. 331). Any response an organism makes to stressors is likely mediated first at the behavioral level and then may have a secondary physiological impact.

A second major challenge to the concept of GAS has focused on its basic tenets of nonspecificity of induction and universal response. The initial arguments for psychosomatic medicine (the influence of psychological factors on health and illness) were based on a specificity approach – different types of illness have different psychological precursors (Alexander and Selesnick, 1966). From this viewpoint, a disease like hypertension is specifically related to difficulty with release of anger, while an illness like asthma is related to exaggerated dependency needs. Although this line of reasoning is generally not considered to have been fruitful (Oken et al., 1962), recent research has demonstrated that there are different patterns of hormonal response to different physical stressors (Mason et al., 1976) and that different kinds of stressing situations may lead to different autonomic responses in a single organism (Lacey, 1967; Shapiro, Tursky, and Schwartz, 1970). Research has also shown that individuals who have historically experienced difficulties with one organ system tend to respond to stressors with signs and symptoms within that system. Wolf and Goodell (1968), for example, found that patients with vascular headache, cardiovascular problems, and duodenal ulcers showed a stress-related hyperactivity in those particular organs. Finally, social situations, emotions, and coping abilities have all been shown to affect different aspects of the stress response.

In general, current research suggests that the stress response is not a simple biological response to nonspecific stressors but rather a complex, interrelated process including the occurrence of a stressor, how it is seen psychologically by the organism, under what circumstances the stressor occurs, how the organism characteristically reacts, and what the resources are that the organism has available for dealing with the stressor. The concept of a general stress reaction may be viable, but only if we assume that it represents the sum of a great many psychological and physiological factors rather than a specific all-or-none response to the occurrence of a stressing event.

This view of stress as a primarily psychological and only secondarily physiological concept has certain implications. First, as already mentioned, the context of a stressor is just as important as the stressor itself in determining whether an organism will respond to the event with stress. Second, psychological characteristics of the organism will also determine the presence or absence and nature of the stress response. Third, while it is true that psychological characteristics of the organism influence the stress response, stressors can themselves be psychological as well as physical. Mason (1968) has pointed out overwhelming evidence of psychological influences on stress-related physiological changes. Only with these factors firmly in mind, then, can we accept the GAS as a basic model for the general nature of the stress response.

STRESS AND ILLNESS

Current interest in the concept of stress as it relates to health and illness undoubtedly began with anecdotal reports of illnesses that seemed to occur during periods of major change in people's lives. For example, it is well known that the recently widowed and divorced have higher mortality rates than all other segments of the population (Carter and Glick, 1970). Adolph Meyer (Lief, 1948) was one of the first to recognize and measure the impact of significant daily life occurrences on subsequent illness. He developed a "life chart" that organized medical, psychological, and sociological data for each individual, and from those charts, patterns began to emerge. Since

that time, many others have investigated the relationship between daily life stressors and illness. The essential point of this
approach is that life events are seen as nonphysical stressors
and that the data suggest there is a positive relationship between those events and the subsequent occurrence of illness.
As might be expected, this relationship is quite complex and its
magnitude appears to be highly dependent on a variety of situational, individual, and constitutional differences.

A simplifed schema of the relationship we have been
discussing may be depicted as follows:

$$\text{STRESSORS} \longrightarrow \text{STRESS} \longrightarrow \text{ILLNESS} \tag{1}$$

This schema outlines a stress pattern that can potentially identify risk factors for the incidence or exacerbation of illness and
provide clues about the most effective way to change the situation (by removing the stressor, by lowering the stress, or by
treating the illness directly). For example, let us suppose an
executive is experiencing a continuing stressor such as constant
job pressure. At this point we could say that he is demon-
strating a stress response that, according to the model of the
GAS, would be in the stage of resistance. Let us suppose that
now an additional stressor occurs, such as exposure to a viral
pathogen. Because our executive is already resisting one stressor, he may well experience sensitization to the second stressor
and succumb to illness more readily than if he were not reacting to a stressor already. Of course, even without an added
stressor our executive might fall ill simply from the effects of
continued pressure from the original stressor. His means of tolerating that stress may well impair his day-to-day functioning
over time and lead to a peptic ulcer, for example.

The foregoing is necessarily an oversimplified version of
current stress-illness research, but it does provide us with a
general introduction to how stress is conceptualized and how it

interacts with illness. Stress is a response, both psychological and biological, that is related to illness according to certain patterns, as predicted by the GAS or other theories we will discuss in the following chapters. Let us now begin to examine the complexity of this relationship from a physiological point of view.

HORMONAL RESPONSES
TO STRESS

THE COMPLEXITY OF HORMONAL STRESS RESPONSES

Selye (1952) initially described the biological stress response as follows: The presence of a stressor (through imperfectly understood mechanisms) acts upon the anterior pituitary and stimulates the secretion of somatotrophic (STH) and adrenocorticotrophic (ACTH) hormones. Although STH acts to stimulate the growth of the body in general, and the growth of thymicolymphatic tissue in particular, it also stimulates the growth of connective tissue to repair physical damage and raises the inflammation potential of the organism to help prevent infiltration by a foreign pathogen. The action of STH can be classified as primarily *prophlogistic,* that is, it augments inflammation and combats the pathogen.

ACTH, on the other hand, stimulates the adrenal cortex to produce two classes of hormones, the mineralocorticoids and the glucocorticoids (Selye, 1952). The mineralocorticoids are classified as prophlogistic corticoids (PC) because they mimic the effect of STH in response to a stressor: they increase inflammation and promote connective tissue proliferation. However, as we noted in Chapter 1, extended prophlogistic reaction – such as a high fever (inflammation reaction) – may threaten the life of the organism. Therefore, if PC action cannot adequately control a stressor, that action must be terminated lest serious consequences result. According to Selye (1956), over-extended prophlogistic activity may cause nephrosclerosis, hypertension, and allergic reactions.

The glucocorticoids are classified as antiphlogistic corticoids (AC) in that they are anti-inflammatory and thus inhibit PC aggrandizement. AC action is initiated as PC-affected tissue becomes increasingly sensitive to the ACs. Selye (1950) called this antiphlogistic response "adaptation." Because ACTH secretion is necessary for AC production, ACTH is generally classified as antiphlogistic. However, continued AC action may also harm the organism as a whole by diminishing specific resistance to microbial pathogens (suppressing the immune response) and delaying wound healing. Other consequences of over-extended antiphlogistic action would be necrosis, thymolysis, adrenal hypertrophy, catabolism, ulcers, and possible precipitation of psychosis (Selye, 1956). In reference to the GAS, PC action would predominate during the alarm reaction and AC action would prevail during the stage of resistance. A graphic representation of Selye's understanding of AC and PC action can be seen in Figure 2. However, in Figure 2, you can see that the stress response is not so simple: a feedback loop serves to regulate ACTH production in the pituitary.

Further research showed that even adrenalectomized animals could demonstrate patterns of resistance to stressors (Selye, 1971), that multiple organ systems were involved in corticoid production, and that autonomic nervous system inputs to the adrenal medulla influenced production of catecholamines (epinephrine and norepinephrine), which, in turn, influenced a wide range of bodily functions such as general metabolism and blood pressure.

Although the effects of epinephrine and norepinephrine interactions in the stress response are not yet completely understood, these catecholamines have been implicated as

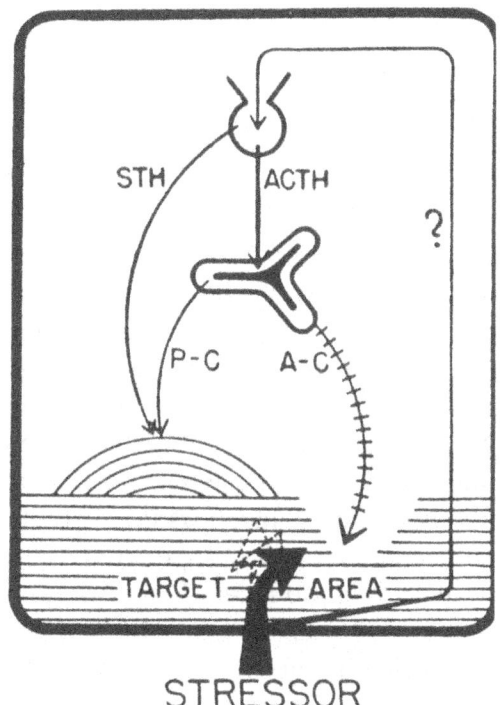

FIGURE 2. Preliminary sketch of stress and inflammation as part of the General Adaptation Syndrome. (From Selye, 1956, p. 106. Reprinted by permission of the McGraw-Hill Book Company.)

contributing to increased risk of heart disease and hypertension (Theorell et al., 1972; Henry, 1976). Palkovits et al. (1975) noted that various stressors in rats produced increased metabolism of norepinephrine in the brain, especially in the medial basal hypothalamus, which is strongly implicated in the pituitary-adrenal stress response. The same authors pointed out that another effect of norepinephrine in the brain was decreased ACTH secretion. Increased norepinephrine metabolism in the brain was also demonstrated in rats that were placed in a situation where they had previously experienced a stressor (shock). The implication of their research is that the norepinephrine metabolism response may be linked with the anticipation of a stressor (Cassens et al., 1980).

On a more behavioral level, Dimsdale and Moss (1980) found, when evaluating public speaking as a stressing experience, that there was a significant difference in the level of epinephrine secreted between the beginning and the middle of a delivered speech. On the other hand, norepinephrine secretion (in plasma) increased during the speech over resting levels, but there was no difference between the beginning and the end of a speech. Thus the authors felt that epinephrine was more sensitive to immediate stressors, while norepinephrine appeared to represent a more stable measure of occurring stress.

The catecholamines, since they appear to react to stressful activity, may reflect behavioral efficiency; presumably, the epinephrine dropped between the beginning and the middle of a speech because the levels of stress decreased as the speaker adapted to the situation. Frankenhauser (1980) found that individuals who tend to secrete more catecholamines—especially epinephrine—performed better in terms of speed and accuracy on various tasks. However, the interaction seems to be even more complex, because this increased efficiency appears to be clearly related to the difficulty of the task. High epinephrine secretors did better than low secretors in monotonous conditions, but in more complex situations—those requiring concentration and discrimination—the high secretors did more poorly. Thus, the role of catecholamines in the stress response has implications for actual pituitary-adrenal responsiveness as well as direct effects on behavior associated with the presence of a stressor.

In addition to the complex relationship of stress to catecholamine secretion, there seem to be specific reactions to specific stressors—for example, hepatic enzyme response to pentobarbital administration (Selye, 1971). Finally, although PC and AC levels were generally recognized as being significantly related to stress, some have advanced the theory that corticoid modes of operation are primarily catalytic in nature rather than directly active (Turner, 1960). Ingle (1954), the major proponent of this point of view, preferred to call the phenomenon the "permissive action" of hormones and contended that these hormones were necessary, although not sufficient, agents in influencing manifestations of stress symptoms.

The details of these interactions are less important to the current discussion than the recognition of their complexity. There may be a gross biological stress reaction that can be measured by pituitary-adrenal functioning, but "it represents a mosaic of numerous local and systemic, humoral and nervous reactions, some of which may protect against one pathogen, others against another" (Selye, 1971, p. 25). It has also been suggested that an individual's constitutional predisposition (for example, through age or sex) to certain hormonal response patterns and reactions to environmental manipulations affects the overall response. Figure 3 represents a more recent, although still simplified, conceptualization of the complexity of the biological stress response. Nevertheless, there is general support for Selye's basic proposition that a large number of stressors effect a general change in pituitary-adrenal activity (Manogue, Leshner, and Candland, 1975).

While the notion of an overall biological stress response remains a valid concept, it is now clear that a great many factors determine that response. Mason et al. (1979) presented one of the most forthright demonstrations of this phenomenon in a study that examined corticosteroid and catecholamine elevations as they related to viral respiratory illness. That adrenal cortical hormones regulate organismic defense systems such as

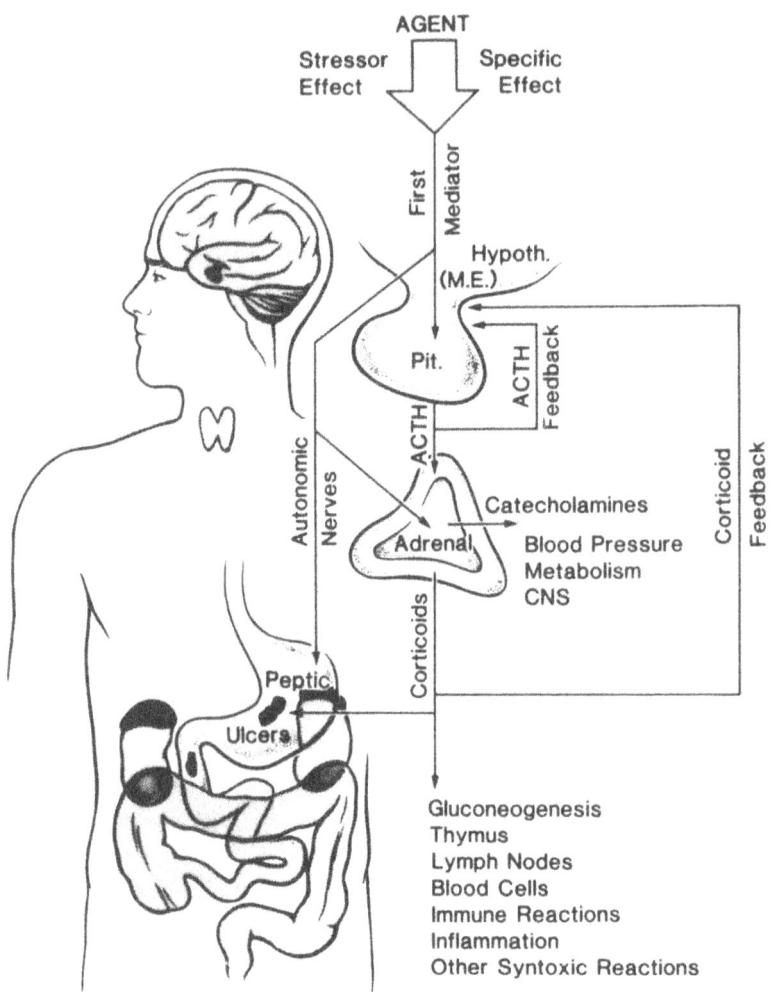

FIGURE 3. Pathways of the Stress Response. (From Selye, 1977, Figure 1, p. 124. Reprinted by permission of *Resident and Staff Physician.*)

lymphocyte production and antibody functioning had been well demonstrated (Dougherty, 1953). Mason examined changes in cortisol production (AC) by measuring seventeen-hydroxycorticosteroid (17-OHCS) excretion in urine in conjunction with catecholamine production before and after onset of fever in viral respiratory illness. In Figure 4, you can see that there was a tendency toward a mild spiking in mean values of 17-OHCS and catecholamines approximately three days prior to the onset of fever. Thus, a specific stressor (virus) activated a general, multifactorial hormonal response even before obvious symptoms occurred.

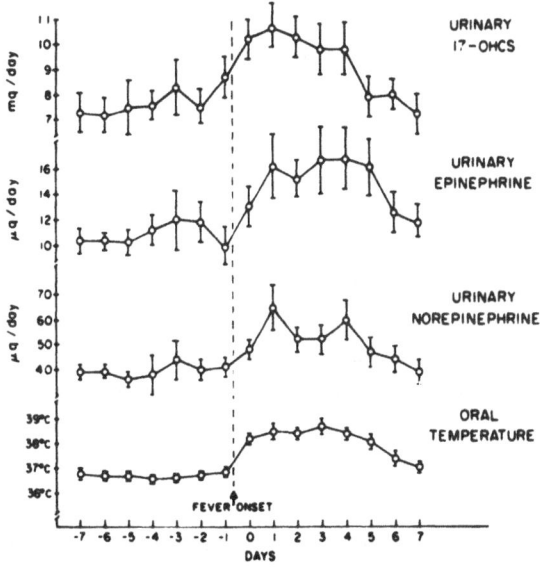

FIGURE 4. Urinary 17-OHCS, epinephrine, norepinephrine and oral temperature levels in relation to onset of acute Adenovirus 4 respiratory illness in Army recruits. (From Mason et al., 1979, Figure 1, p. 24. Reprinted by permission of Opinion Publications, Inc., and the author.)

PSYCHOLOGICAL INFLUENCES ON HORMONAL RESPONSES

The influence of psychological factors on stress-related hormonal patterns has been well documented. Early on, Hill et al. (1956) described a significant relationship between 17-OHCS concentration in urine and ACTH production in response to psychological stressors in man. Bliss, Migeon, Branch, and Samuels (1956) further refined the method of 17-OHCS analysis in urine and concluded that stressing life situations consistently increased 17-OHCS urine levels. Mason and Brady (1956) found a significant association between plasma 17-OHCS levels and conditioned emotional responses in monkeys.

Gradually, these earlier findings became more refined. Mason (1959a; 1959b) measured 17-OHCS levels in monkeys under varied housing conditions, location transfers, and handling and venipuncture. Mason found that plasma 17-OHCS levels were positively related to the "first experience" of novel stimuli, conditioned avoidance (learning how to avoid a noxious situation), conditioned emotional response (anticipating a noxious situation by reacting to a learned warning sign such as a bell or light), and punishment. Seventeen-hydroxycorticosteroid levels were negatively related to weekend rest periods. In the same studies, Mason assayed 17-OHCS excretion in the urine of human subjects during sleep deprivation experiments and in air force pilots on a prolonged nonstop flight and found increased levels of 17-OHCS in both of the groups that he examined. Mason also studied pre-operative surgical patients and found high correlations between plasma 17-OHCS and psychological test responses to be indicative of general anxiety.

Seventeen-hydroxycorticosteroid levels in the plasma and urine of college students have been shown to be significantly related to examination stressors. Bliss, Migeon, Branch, and Samuels (1956) found significant plasma 17-OHCS elevations in medical students before a final examination. Venning, Dyren-furth, and Beck (1957) and Hodges, Jones, and Stockham (1962) reported similar results for urinary and plasma 17-OHCS measures in general college students before final examinations. These studies of naturally occurring stressors confirmed the reactivity of the biological stress response in everyday life.

Studies that have attempted to experimentally induce stress in humans have also generally supported the theories concerning 17-OHCS production in response to stressors. Hetzel, Schottstaedt, Grace, and Wolff (1955), using a stressing inter-view technique, found that elevated 17-OHCS levels in urine were produced when topics of significance to the interviewees were discussed. Handlon et al. (1962) and Wadeson, Mason, Hamburg, and Handlon (1963) reported that groups of subjects responded to war movies with significant plasma 17-OHCS elevations but experienced a marked decrease in plasma 17-OHCS levels while viewing Walt Disney nature films. Mason (1968, p. 592) summarized this variety of evidence and con-cluded that: "In general, then, studies with human subjects pro-vide almost unanimous support for the conclusion that 17-OHCS levels sensitively reflect psychological influences."

Nevertheless, it has also been demonstrated that an in-dividual can modify a response as specific as 17-OHCS. Tecce, Friedman, and Mason (1966) studied twenty parents of children with leukemia and found an inverse, significant relationship between amount of psychological defensiveness and urinary 17-OHCS. Psychological observation of these parents sug-gested that they were not dealing effectively with the stressing agent of their child's disease. In related research, Wolff, Fried-man, Hofer, and Mason (1964) and Wolff, Hofer, and Mason (1964) used extensive interview data, 17-OHCS urinary excre-tion levels, and predictive and postdictive data over periods of two years to determine how effective psychological defenses are against the long-term stress of having a child with diagnosed leukemia. In general, they found that "the more *effectively* a parent defends against the threat of loss, the lower will be his 17-OHCS excretion rate" (Wolff, Hofer, and Mason, 1964, p. 592). "Effectiveness" of defenses referred to the "immediate success of tension reduction by the defense." The degree to which these defenses were effective was a reflection of the chronic individual differences in the parents who were studied. Poe, Rose, and Mason (1970) further supported the hypothesis that psychological defenses diminish stress response. They used forty-six army recruits to study the relationship between 17-OHCS urinary excretion and psychological ratings. They examined profile characteristics on a personality test, the Minnesota Multiphasic Personality Inventory (MMPI, see Dahlstrom, Welsh, and Dahlstrom, 1972), and the experience of environmental events for those recruits who fell into the upper and lower quartiles of 17-OHCS levels and concluded that: "what defines an effective defense, as judged by 17-OHCS excretion, is not the type of defense, nor solely one's *defensive ability,* but an interaction between one's usual modes of psychological defenses diminish stress response. They used defended against" (Poe, Rose, and Mason, 1970, pp. 376–377). The importance of psychological factors in modifying biological stress response is thus widely recognized and will be discussed in more detail in the next chapter.

Because it has always been difficult to compare complex hormonal measurements with detailed psychological measurements, the bulk of studies examining relationships between psychological stressors and biological response have tended to compare the hormonal responses of "stressed" groups with "non-stressed" groups of individuals. This research approach is rather weak, since individuals differ in their constitutional predisposition and makeup, and the exact nature, magnitude, and timing of their stress response will also differ. A thorough, long-term systematic study of hormonal responses to stressors was conducted by Ursin, Baade, and Levine (1978) and deserves extended mention here. They examined stress response in parachute trainees over a two-month period, conducting a detailed examination of the presence of psychological stressors (parachute training), individual perceptions of the stressors (psychological measures), and biological stress response (hormonal and other physiological measures). Ursin et al. took basal measures before parachute training began and then measured again before and after training on successive days that the trainees jumped from a tower to simulate parachute drops. In general, the results demonstrated that psychological measures of fear (as an index of perceived stressors) declined on successive jump days as the individuals became more accustomed to jumping; this was directly related to declines in levels of cortisol (AC), catecholamines, and free fatty acids circulating in the bloodstream. However, plasma testosterone (a gonadotropic hormone) and blood glucose levels, although initially following the same pattern, eventually returned to basal levels. (See Figures 5, 6, and 7 for examples of these changes.)

The complexity of these psychological and physiological changes is further illustrated by the fact that they do not vary independently of each other; note the correlations between various hormones illustrated in Figure 8. Overall, the authors found that while there was a general increase in psychological and physiological measures of fear when parachute training began, those measurements gradually decreased once the trainees had adequately mastered their tasks. If performance was not adequate or if measures of psychological defensiveness remained high, cortisol activation also remained high—a finding consistent with the interaction between psychological defensiveness and 17-OHCS production in the parents of children dying from leukemia. Thus, the importance of *coping* is introduced as another variable in the stress-illness paradigm:

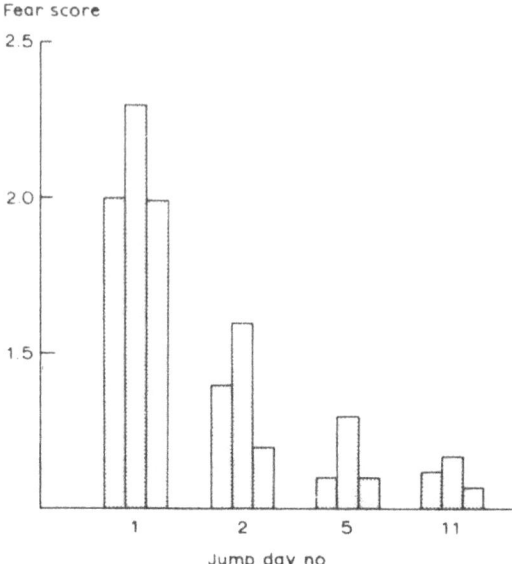

FIGURE 5. Self-rating of fear by men in parachute tower training. The three columns for jump represent the average scores at the bottom of the tower, those just before jumping, and those just after the jump. (From Ursin et al., 1978, Figure 4.1, p. 44. Reprinted by permission of Academic Press and the author.)

"Coping, by our definition, occurred when there was a response decrement in the physiological activation processes accompanying the response to threat" (Ursin, Baade, and Levine, 1978, p. 214).

The biological stress response is psychologically determined not only by the appraisal of a stressor (measure of fear), but also by an ameliorative factor (successful coping). In other words, the stress is no longer treated as a stressor when it can be dealt with adequately. If there is no longer a stressor, then the progression to the stress response and the subsequent manifestation of illness are circumvented. The paradigm that was

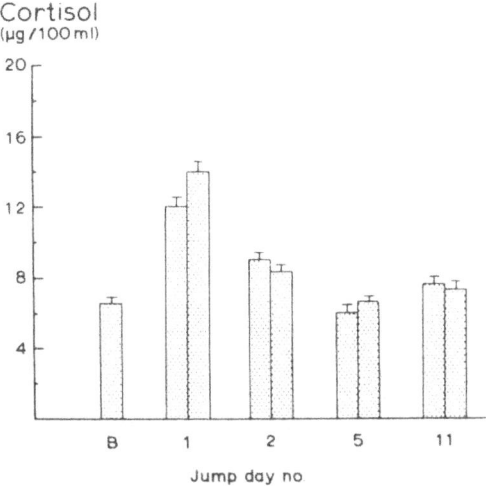

FIGURE 6. Plasma levels of cortisol, B basal level of men in parachute training. For each jump day, two samples were obtained, one immediately after the jump and one 20 minutes later. The vertical line on the top of each bar indicates the standard error. (From Ursin et al., 1978, Figure 6.1, p. 54. Reprinted by permission of Academic Press and the author.)

presented in Chapter 1 can now be expanded to include the coping response as it interacts with the stressor to determine the biological stress response:

$$STRESSOR \longrightarrow STRESS \longrightarrow COPING$$

Unsuccessful $\longrightarrow$ ILLNESS   (2)

Successful

This model suggests that with the onset of a perceived stressor, an initial biological reaction occurs. If nothing is done to deal with the stressor or if dealing with the stressor is ineffective it can be expected that the stressor may eventually result in ill-

21

Testosterone
(ng/ml)

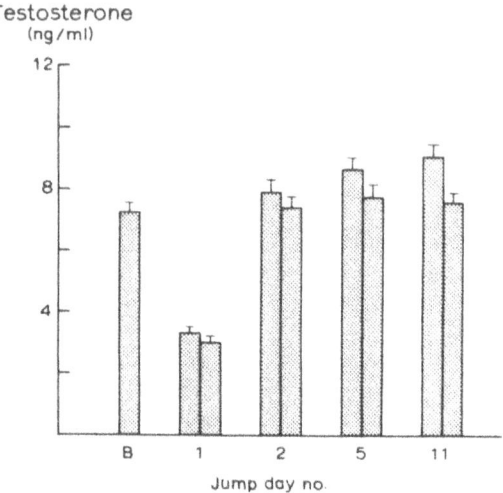

Jump day no.

FIGURE 7.   Plasma testosterone levels of men in parachute training. (From Ursin et al., 1978, Figure 6.1, p. 59. Reprinted by permission of Academic Press and the author.)

ness. However, if coping is effective, it either ameliorates or nullifies the stressor, the biological response is diminished, and, consequently, the risk of illness is decreased.

IMPLICATIONS FOR ILLNESS

At this point in our discussion, it may be premature to speculate on how specifically the stress response affects illness. Some direct effects described by Selye (1956), such as ulceration, have already been mentioned. In an even broader statement, Baxter and Rousseau (1979) concluded that glucocorticoids (cortisol) initially suppress every phase of immunologic and inflammatory response. We will discuss these effects more thoroughly in Chapter 7. For the moment, let us consider one of the elements of the stress response that Ursin et al. (1978)

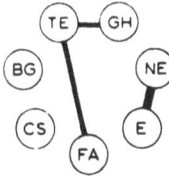

BASAL

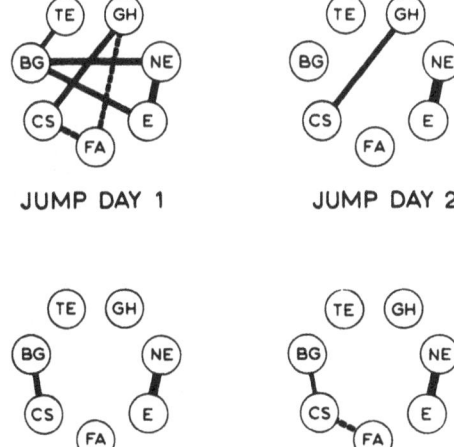

JUMP DAY 1   JUMP DAY 2

JUMP DAY 5   JUMP DAY 11

FIGURE 8. Correlations between plasma and urine variables for the basal day and for post-jump values of catecholamines and the other variables from the second blood samples. TE, testosterone; GH, growth hormone, NE, norepinephrine; E, epinephrine; FA, free fatty acids; CS, cortisol; BG, blood glucose. (From Ursin et al., 1978, Figure 12.1, p. 109. Reprinted by permission of Academic Press and the author.)

described: the mobilization of fatty acids when a stressor is initially presented. As the authors pointed out, increased fatty acid circulation over extended periods could lead to atherosclerosis (Carlson, 1970), cardiac arrhythmias (Oliver, 1974), and coronary artery disease (Westlund and Nicolaysen, 1972). Thus, failure to adequately cope with a stressor for a length of time could increase the risk of developing these illnesses.

Let us reconsider the case of the pressured executive discussed in Chapter 1. As you recall, it was suggested that if a stress response were to continue, the executive might be subject to crossed sensitization effects and also to direct stress illness effects. The example of fatty acid mobilization over extended periods would demonstrate such direct effects if the individual could not effectively cope with a present stressor. However, if he could successfully cope, the stress response would not continue and his vulnerability would cease. The biological stress response is thus truly related to psychological factors in both a perceptual and a reactionary sense. The body will react to a stressor only if the stressor is perceived as such; even so, stress will cease or diminish if the stressor is dealt with effectively. Let us now explore the psychological aspects of the biological stress response more thoroughly.

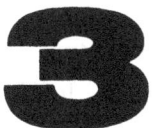

COGNITIVE FACTORS
IN STRESS

APPRAISING AND COPING WITH STRESSORS

An event can be a stressor for one person and not for another. For example, the death of a parent may be a tragedy for a child who had a strong and positive relationship with the parent, while that same death may be a relief to an adult who has had an unpleasant and demanding relationship with the deceased as an employer. From a psychological perspective, the study we discussed in Chapter 2 (Mason et al., 1976) demonstrated that even forced situations generally regarded as stressing, such as extreme heat, cold, or fasting, did not result in a physiological stress response in the monkey subjects if psychological factors were controlled effectively. In humans, the perception of stressors is necessarily even more complex, in that any stressor has psychological characteristics and the individual perception of that stressor will depend on the context of the stressor, the context of the individual, past experience with the stressor, and how successfully the individual can cope with the stressor.

Wolf and Goodell (1968) have suggested that cultural bias, work-related impact, and a sense of personal and social vulnerability are factors that lead to the recognition (or ascription) of threat for any given stimulus. They described response to a stressor as an adaptive reaction that may or may not be of long-term benefit to the individual. Lazarus (1977) refined this notion, focusing on the cognitive appraisal made when an individual perceives a stimulus as a threat. From this appraisal of threat flows an emotional response that includes the appraisal itself, physiological changes, and some activity that is both instrumental (it does something about the stressor) and expressive (it produces an affective reaction). In a simplified sense, for a stimulus to be stressing it must be perceived as such. Lazarus (1977, pp. 147–148) described some of the factors involved in determining how stimuli are perceived:

> Consider two different persons who perceive that they are facing a demand, or the juxtaposition of several demands, which seem to them to be at the borderline or beyond their capacity to master—too much is expected of them. As a result of their individual histories and particular personalities, Person A feels that failure of mastery reflects his own inadequacy, while Person B, by contrast, feels the same pressure but interprets the situation as one in which people are constantly trying to use and abuse him. Both experience similar degrees of anticipatory stress and are mobilized to cope with the problem. Prior to the confrontation with the dangerous situation, both experience anxiety, and anticipatory emotion produced by appraised threat. In Person A, the anxiety is mixed with depression, while in Person B, the anxiety is mixed with external blaming and anger. Following the confrontation in which both perform badly, Person A will experience mainly loss and depression, while Person B mainly anger and resentment. Thus a similar set of overwhelming demands has been construed or appraised quite differently by these two individuals. If, on the other hand, these persons do well in the confrontation, one may experience more elation than the other, depending on whether the explanation of the success is luck or their own perseverance and skill. In any case, such subtle dif-

ferences in appraisal of a stress commerce with the environment underlie variations among individuals in the severity (and possibly pattern) of bodily reactions.

How an individual deals with the perception of a stressor is what we call the "coping process." In the work of Ursin et al. (1978), described in Chapter 2, coping was seen as the mastery of a threatening task – parachute jumping. Lazarus et al. (1980) further extended the definition of the coping process to include individual psychological effectiveness that either increases or decreases the risk of maladaptive illness. For example, if a person reacts to a stressing situation by increased smoking, drinking, or overeating, or is predisposed to try and control any type of stressor he comes in contact with, his risk of illness will be increased. Lazarus and his coworkers, like Mason (1971), concluded that the essential mediator of the stress response is psychological and that the cognitive appraisal of threat is all-important to the initiation of the response. The success or failure of the coping process will determine whether the stress response will be relaxed or maintained.

An example of the Lazarus et al. (1980) approach to appraisal and coping has been demonstrated in a study by Aldrich and Mendkoff (1963). They found that when aged individuals were displaced and moved to another living situation, such as a nursing home or a child's home, higher incidence of mortality occurred. However, the mortality rate evidently differs depending on how each aged individual copes with the displacement; those who reacted with psychosis or depression tended to do poorly, while those who responded angrily or philosophically to the change tended to do better.

Among the classic demonstrations of the importance of cognitive appraisal and coping in mediating stress and illness are some experiments performed by Brady and by Weiss. Back in

1950, Selye had found a positive relationship between the oc-currence of peptic and duodenal ulcers in humans and emo-tional stressors such as war or the "increase in the stressors and stress of modern life." Brady (1958), in a series of well-detailed experiments, produced gastrointestinal lesions in Rhesus monkeys by subjecting them to the psychological stressor of shock avoidance. The essential design of these experiments was to have two monkeys paired together, with both of them receiving an electrical shock if a bar was not pressed at certain intervals. However, only one monkey in the pair was able to press the bar; the other monkey was a passive partner. The monkey responsible for pressing the bar (the "executive" monkey) developed more gastrointestinal lesions than his passive partner. Brady felt that this demonstrated the stressor characteristics of vigilance and decision making on the part of the executive monkey, since both monkeys received the same number of shocks over time.

The paradigm turned out not to be so simple. Weiss (1970) yoked two rats together in a similar experiment. Neither rat had control over when the shocks would occur, but one rat's shocks were preceded by a warning signal and the other rat's were not. The rats who were not warned of the oncoming shock developed six times the number of stomach lesions found in the rats that were warned. Thus, predictability of an oncoming stressor appeared to be a significant variable in ill-ness symptoms associated with a stressor. Weiss (1972) went on to examine what happened when the subject *could* control the stressor onset. Again, rats were yoked together, but this time one rat was able to rotate a wheel and avoid shock when a signal light came on. The second rat had similar access to a wheel but could do nothing in terms of avoiding shock, and a third rat was used as a control, receiving the same warning signal but no shocks. Figure 9 shows the number of stomach le-sions in the three groups of subjects. The rat that received no

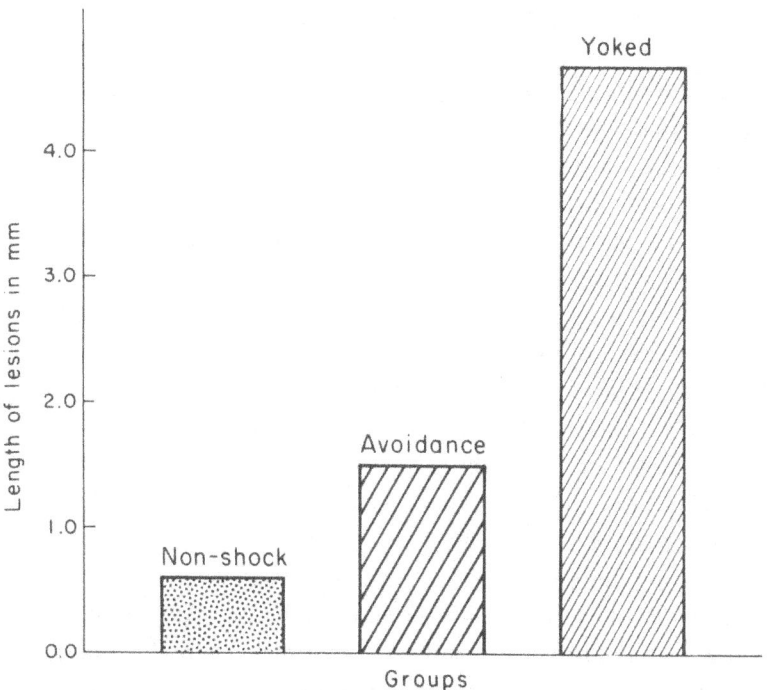

FIGURE 9. Effect of being able to perform an avoidance coping response on the amount of stomach lesions. Each yoked rat received exactly the same electric shocks as his avoidance partner because the electrodes on their tails were wired in series. (From Miller, 1980, in *Selye's Guide to Stress Research*, vol. 1, Hans Selye, M.D., ed., © 1980 by Hans Selye, M.D. Figure 7.6, p. 145. Reprinted by permission of Van Nostrand Reinhold Company.)

shocks had the fewest lesions; the rat that was able to control the shocks had more; but the greatest number of lesions appeared in the animal that received shocks but was unable to control their occurrence. Thus, control over an oncoming stressor was shown to be an important variable in coping.

You may be wondering how Brady's findings (1958), where control of a stressor was associated with increased gastrointestinal lesions, compare to the results of Weiss (1970, 1972) where predictability and control of a stressor resulted in decreased lesions. At least a partial answer to this paradox was provided by Tsuda and Hirai (1975), who demonstrated in an experiment similar to Weiss's that the difficulty of the coping task was quite important. If the response required of the animal was simple, such as pressing a bar or turning a wheel one time after the warning stimulus occurred, the coping rats had fewer stomach lesions than their yoked partners. However, if the task was more difficult, such as having to press the bar many times after the warning, the coping rats had more stomach lesions than their yoked partners. The task used by Brady (1958) was more difficult in that it did not provide clear warning stimuli, but rather demanded a continuous action on the part of the ex-executive monkey over time to avoid shock. Thus, although predictability and control are important variables in the stress response (and in subsequent illness), they also interact with the complexity of the task required for coping with the stressor. Predictability and control in face of complex stressors may well be less adaptive than having no control.

Let us look again at Aldrich and Mendkoff's (1963) study about the effects of changes in residence on health among the elderly. Those who were able to deal with their change in life philosophically (that is, by resigning themselves to the situation) fared better than those who could not; change of residence was a significant stressor they could do little about, no matter what they preferred. On the other hand, in the study by Ursin et al. (1978), stress was lessened for individuals who mastered the task at hand (coped); they were able to control the stressor effectively in ways that eventually became simple or second nature to them.

An important aspect of this interaction between the nature of a stressor and the factors of predictability and coping has been pointed out by Miller (1980). In reviewing a number of experiments by Seligman (1975), Miller discovered that if animals were exposed to a number of tasks where they were subjected to stressors, such as shock, in which they had no control and were unable to avoid the stressor, a curious behavior developed—the animal seemed to give up and do nothing. Seligman termed this behavior "learned helplessness." In effect, the animal does nothing because past experience suggests that there is nothing it *can* do in face of the stressor. Miller pointed to clinical evidence that patients with chronic illness, such as inoperable cancer, fare worse over the short run if they give up; that is, they "turn their face to the wall and soon die for no apparent reason." The phenomenon of "giving up" is well known among medical practitioners as an indicator of a poor prognosis in any serious illness (Schmale, 1972). It does not take much of a logical jump to recognize that a person's history of successful and unsuccessful coping with stressors, dating back to childhood, will have a significant impact on how he or she appraises the threat of a stressor and copes with it. Thus, the ability to learn new ways of coping is crucial in meeting the threat of different stressors in the course of a lifetime.

Let us stop for a moment and review the complex cognitive factors we are dealing with in stress responses. Whether a stressor is seen as such depends in part on what experience the individual has had in the past coping with that stressor, as well as how the individual has learned to cope in general. If the stressor is perceived as threatening, the individual's ability to cope with it is related, in part, to his success at doing so in the past. However, the perceived magnitude of the stressor will also be directly related to the kind of coping behavior required; the larger the stressor and the more complex the required coping response, the more serious the health effects of attempting to deal with the problem directly. The smaller the stressor and the more simple the necessary response, the more effective coping behaviors will be in avoiding illness. The experiments we have discussed so far have focused on laboratory animals; with people, the interactions will necessarily be more complex. The magnitude of the stressor will not depend solely on how large a shock is, but rather on how the stressor is perceived by the individual. How simple a coping response is perceived to be will depend on past experience and the ability to learn ways of dealing with the situation at hand. For one person, facing a complex mathematical problem will not seem difficult, either because he has dealt with such problems successfully in the past or because he has learned the coping responses necessary, such as appropriate formulas or computer techniques that make solving the problem easy. For someone else, without such past experience or skills, the magnitude of the stressor would be much larger and coping responses would necessarily be more complex. The old adage that sometimes it may be better to leave a situation than to attempt to change it is borne out by our current understanding of the stress response.

Antonovsky (1979) has expanded on the interactions we have just examined from a different point of view that deserves mention. He saw coping as a tension-reduction mechanism. A stressor, by his definition, is a demand that taxes or exceeds the resources of the system. Tension is the response to that stressor, while stress itself is the reaction when one has failed to reduce that tension. According to Antonovsky (1979, p. 73), the tension-reduction response is an omnipresent factor in everyday life, since "the overwhelming number of human beings are, most of the time, in the throes of confronting what they define as stressors." He argued that we should be concerned not with how an individual's perceptions or lack of coping lead to stress and illness, but rather with how effectively an individual can maintain health; salutogenesis (the promotion of health), not pathogenesis (the development of disease), should be our focus. This distinction is important because generally, most of us perceive stressors accurately (in terms of our own lives) and deal with them effectively most of the time. It is only when something goes awry in an otherwise well-functioning system that stress and illness occur. Stress is thus seen as a residual factor from a failed attempt to deal with a stressor. Antonovsky saw successful salutogenesis as a "sense of coherence" that is based on the extent to which a person feels confident that his internal and external environments are predictable and that things will work out as well as can be expected. This point of view echoes earlier assessments of the importance of effective psychological defenses in dealing with stressors made by Hofer et al. (1972) as well as the importance of differing emotional reactions stressed by Lazarus (1977).

A MODEL OF COMPLEX PSYCHOLOGICAL INTERACTION

Rahe and Arthur (1978) have presented a model of the interaction of a stressful life event, its appraisal, and the reaction to it in terms of effects on illness (see Figure 10). The first part of their model—the perception of the stressor—is depicted as a "polarizing filter." This is the lens through which we see the world; it is determined by our past experiences and perceived personal and interpersonal resources. The next step in the model depicts how our psychological defenses respond to those perceptions, for example, by denial, distortion, or acceptance. Based on how these defenses interact with our perceptions, in step 3 psychophysiological responses take place, ranging from bodily symptoms (such as headaches), which symbolically represent a denied stressor, to physiological responses (such as elevated lipids), which are a bodily reaction to an acknowledged stressor. In the next step, the individual tries to eliminate the physiological response by such measures as taking medications, increasing exercise, or moving away from the stressor. If the stress-reduction activities are ineffective, illness-related behavior takes place (step 5), such as seeking medical

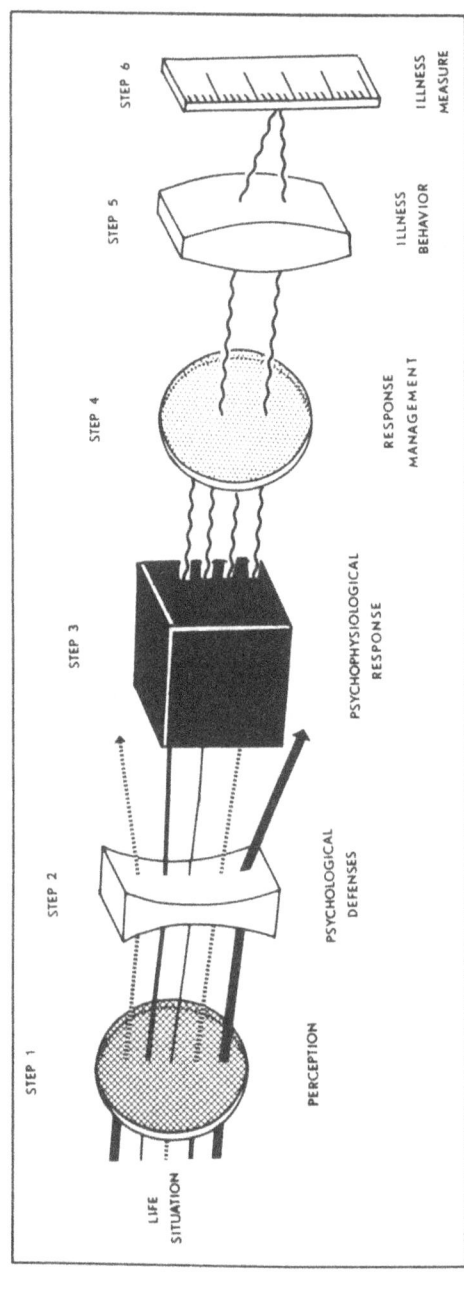

FIGURE 10. A model of interaction in stress and illness. (From Rahe and Arthur, 1978, Figure 1, p. 7. Reprinted by permission of Opinion Publications, Inc., and the author.)

help or missing work. The final step of the model depicts how the clinician or the researcher measures the illness by taking blood pressure, making a medical diagnosis, or using some other method.

Although this model cannot fully account for the myriad of factors affecting the response to a stressor or fully explain the related implications for illness, it illustrates well the complexity that makes it difficult to clearly delineate the steps between the onset of a stressor and ensuing illness. Beyond the factors that have already been shown to affect this relationship, social supports (which will be treated in the next chapter) and the complexity of individual personalities (which will be treated in another book in this series) are also important. In a summary review of which individuals are seen by researchers as best suited to deal with stressors, Chan (1977) concluded that individuals with high self-esteem, internal orientation, and freedom from intense anxiety are most able to manifest positive and adaptive responses to stressors.

At this point in our discussion, the paradigm we have been working with in summarizing the relationship between stressor and illness might best be represented as follows:

$$STRESSOR \longrightarrow APPRAISAL \longrightarrow STRESS \longrightarrow COPING$$

$$\begin{array}{ll} \text{Unsuccessful} \longrightarrow \text{ILLNESS} & (3) \\ \text{Successful} \end{array}$$

The key to this model is that it may be modified by individual appraisal and by individual coping effectiveness. In addition, as mentioned in earlier parts of this book, the stress response takes time to develop, whether you follow the GAS schema or some other model. For illness to develop, the stress response must also be present for some time.

The implications of the research reviewed in these last two chapters are that a stressor leads to stress and that stress leads to illness only if nothing is done about the stressor or if what is done is ineffective. Given that stressors confront us all and that the majority of us tend to be more or less healthy, perhaps Antonovsky's (1979) theory is correct and what we need to be concerned with is not how stress leads to illness, but why, in some cases, our general ability to maintain health gives way under stress.

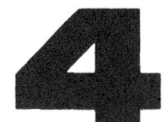

SOCIAL MEDIATORS OF
THE STRESS RESPONSE

THE IMPORTANCE OF SOCIAL SUPPORT

Although individual differences in appraisal of stressors and coping styles are extremely important in determining relationships between stress and illness, the social context of the individual and his perceived social support are also major contributing factors. For example, although bereavement has been linked to an increased risk of mortality, how one deals with the bereavement may significantly modify this risk. Maddison and Walker (1967), using widows' subjective reports of physical and mental health, found that those who had "bad outcomes" (increased illness) perceived their social networks as failing to meet their needs and being actively unhelpful. Thus, the resources we have discussed as being perceived as available in terms of the appraisal of stressors and in terms of coping responses are not only individual but also social in nature.

What are some of the social supports we are discussing? An obvious one is a family relationship, such as marriage. Chiriboga and Dean (1978) identified a relationship between marital difficulties and psychological disturbance symptoms. More generally, Caplan (1974) defined social support as including enduring interpersonal ties to a group sharing similar status and values that can be depended on to provide emotional support, help, and physical resources and to give needed feedback. Such groups may be found at home in the family, at work, at church, or in other social settings.

Kiritz and Moos (1974), in a review of the literature, attempted to further define the dimensions of social networks that might tend to exacerbate stress. The first dimension they identified was a relationship dimension; in general, they suggested that when interpersonal strife occurs, high levels of personal involvement with others can lead to an increased stress response (physiologically measured). A second dimension centered on personal development and included a sense of responsibility and commitment toward surrounding events. Higher responsibility leads to a greater stress response when difficulties arise, for example, in work-related activities. This dimension appears to relate to the factors of decision making and control (Brady, 1958; Weiss, 1972) discussed in Chapter 3. The third dimension that Kiritz and Moos described was concerned with change versus stability in surrounding interpersonal systems. Greater change leads to greater stress.

Another approach to evaluating the effects of social interactions on stress has been to observe the effects of general social change on symptoms of illness. Long ago, Faris and Dunham (1939) realized that the incidence of medical and psychiatric disorders was higher in deteriorating urban areas. Rabkin and Streuning (1976) later noted that although the effects of stressors may be reduced for people with effective social networks (as suggested by Kiritz and Moos, 1974), they will be exacerbated by deficiencies or impairments in those networks. Rabkin and Streuning identified three categories of deficiencies in social systems: social isolation, marginality (minority membership), and status inconsistency. Social isolation means being alone and not being involved with others. Uninvolved people are more vulnerable to a variety of chronic diseases. Minority membership means belonging to a low-status group or a group with few members compared to the size of surrounding groups. Rabkin and Streuning pointed out that ethnic density (the number of people in a group) is inversely related to psychiatric hospitalization rates. Status inconsistency exists when a person occupies two or more distinct roles that have incompatible social aspects. For example, there might be a lack of fit between education and occupation, between sex and employment, or between education and financial status. Hinkle (1974), in study of semiskilled telephone workers, found that the healthiest subjects were from families whose aspirations and interests coincided with their present occupational status. He found that workers who were frequently ill, on the other hand, tended to come from families with educational or social status levels inappropriately high for the type of work being done.

In a study of specific illnesses, Kasl et al. (1979) found that West Point cadets who were at risk for infectious mononucleosis due to evidence of the development of an antibody to the Epstein-Barr virus ran a higher risk for developing clinical symptoms of the disease if they: (1) had fathers who were overachievers, (2) had a high level of motivation, and (3) were doing poorly academically. These risk factors also significantly affected the length of hospitalization for the illness once it occurred.

These dimensions of social interaction, however, are not clearly independent of a more general factor mentioned at the start of this chapter: social support. Although Kiritz and Moos found layoffs of workers to be related to increased health changes, Cobb (1974), who identified job responsibility and system change as also important in health changes related to being laid off, found that physical changes were remarkably different depending on the degree of social support workers experienced at their time of crisis. Strong social support resulted in fewer physical symptoms. An even more classic example of the importance of social support was illustrated by Swank (1949), who reported that in wartime, previously healthy soldiers began to experience combat fatigue regularly after about 65 percent of their companions had become casualties.

Several people have clarified the nature of the interaction between stress and social support. Nuckolls, Cassel, and Kaplan (1972) measured psychosocial assets and stressing life events in relation to prognosis for a normal pregnancy. Assets were first measured early in pregnancy and then life stressors were measured for the two years preceding pregnancy and at 32 weeks into the pregnancy in order to see what changes had occurred. Alone, neither social assets nor life changes could determine a tendency toward complications in pregnancy. Together, however, if life changes were high before or during pregnancy, women with high social assets had only one-third the rate of complications found in women with lower social assets. An interactive effect appears important here. Cassel (1975) suggested that deficiencies in support systems do not contribute to illness in and of themselves unless stress is present. When strong support systems are available, stressors have only a minor impact.

The interaction between life stressors and social support has been further described in a model proposed by Dean and Lin (1977). Essentially, this model suggests that stressing life events have a positive relationship with illness, while social support is negatively related to illness. Lin, Simeone, Ensel, and Kuo (1979) tested this model to determine how these two aspects interact in a more detailed way. They found that social support appears to be an effective buffer against specific illness symptoms, independent of the occurrence of stressing life events, although stressing events are also significantly related to illness. They concluded that social support is just as important, if not more so, than the stressing events themselves, and the effects of both are probably additive in nature.

The weight of the evidence suggests that there is a clear relationship between social support and illness. That relationship may have independent characteristics, but it clearly plays a mediating role that can significantly modify any interaction between a stressor, stress, and illness.

A GENERAL INTEGRATION

Jenkins (1979) evaluated the importance of social supports during life stress in terms of adequacy of social skills among individuals. In his study of a group of air-traffic controllers, he found a strong association between general life stressors and psychological problems in controllers who had below-average social coping resources. Jenkins did more than evaluate the importance of interpersonal resources; he also attempted to integrate those resources with biological, psychological (cognitive), and sociocultural aspects of the way various types of illness outcomes relate to stress. Jenkins' attempt at integration (shown in Table 1) was based, in large part, on Selye's concept of the GAS. The *alarm reaction* is similar to Selye's concept, the *defensive reaction* is much like Selye's stage of resistance, and the *pathological end-state* is analagous to Selye's stage of exhaustion. However, Jenkins expanded on the concepts that were presented in Chapter 3, focusing on how interaction with stress can be adaptive or maladaptive (producing health or illness). Table 2 illustrates Jenkins' attempts to broaden the integration of the individual and interpersonal aspects of stressor appraisal and coping ability that we have already discussed. While many of the factors listed in this table are not vital to the purpose of this volume, they do illustrate, again, the complexity of our subject. In the model, adaptive capacity refers to the resources available to the individual for perceiving stressors and learning to cope with them. The incredible variety of stressors that can affect an individual are also well described.

TABLE 1
FIVE ASPECTS OF THE INTERACTION OF STRESS AND THE ORGANISM

Class of Variable	Example Associated with Health	Example Associated with Disease
Adaptive Capacity (Host Resistance)	Problem-solving skills Ego Strength	Inexperience Copelessness
Stimulus Input ("Stressor")	Mild, superficial Brief	Intense, Invasive Prolonged
Alarm Reaction (Immediate Distress)	Appropriate to stimulus Used as a cue to action	Inappropriate in amount, kind, or interpretation
Defensive Reaction (Resistance, Adjustment)	Adaptive defense reduces stressor	Maladaptive defense fails to reduce stressor or creates "side effect"
Pathological End-State (Disease, Decompensation)	Prevented by Adaptive Capacity or Adequate Defense	Reduced level of function or structural change

(From Jenkins, 1979, Table 1, p. 5. Reprinted by permission of Opinion Publications, Inc., and the author.)

Table 2
A MODEL DEPICTING THE INTERACTION OF STRESS AND THE ORGANISM

	Adaptive Capacity	Stressors	Alarm Reaction	Defensive Reaction	Pathological End-State
Biological Level	State of physique, nutrition, vigor Natural or acquired immunities	Deprivation of biological needs Excess inputs of physical or biological agents	Arousal — hunger, thirst, pain, fatigue Changes in physiological function	General adaptation syndrome Physiological compensation Shifts in metabolism Changes in pain threshold	Deficiency diseases "Exhaustion" Addictions Chronic dysfunction Structural damage
Psychological Level	Resourcefulness, problem solving ability Ego Strength Flexibility Social skills	Perceptions and interpretations of danger, threat, loss, disappointment, frustration, or sense of failure or hopelessness Loss of self-acceptance Threat to security	Feeling of deprivation — boredom, grief, sadness Feelings of anxiety, pressure, guilt Fear of danger	Ego defenses — denial, repression, projection Defensive neuroses Perceptual defenses — wishes, fantasies, motives Planning Problem solving	Despair, apathy Chronic personality pattern disturbances Psychoses Chronic affective disorders Meaninglessness
Interpersonal Level	Primary relationships including family Network of social supports	Social isolation Lack of acceptance Insults, punishments, rejections Changes in social groups, especially losses	Antagonism, conflict, suspicion Feelings of rejection, punishment	Defensive, rigid social relating Avoidance Assuming sick role Aggressiveness "Acting out" Enlisting social supports	Chronic exploitation Becoming an outcast Imprisonment Permanent disruption of interpersonal ties Chronic failure to fulfill roles
Sociocultural Level	Values Norms and practices "Therapeutic" social institutions Systems of knowledge and technology	Cultural change Role conflict Status incongruity Value conflicts with important others Forced change in life situation	Communication of concern and alarm Expressive behavior of crowds Mobilization of social structures	Culturally prescribed defenses — scapegoating prejudice Explanatory ideologies Legal and moral system Use of curers and institutions	Alienation, anomie Breakdown of social order Disintegration of the cultural systems of values and norms

(From Jenkins, 1979, Table 2, p. 6. Reprinted by permission of Opinion Publications, Inc., and the author.)

The wide range of individual differences and their relationship to illness and health are treated in another volume in this series (Bieliauskas, 1981), as is the equally broad topic of sociocultural influences on health and illness (Counte and Christman, 1981).

We can now complete the modification of our expanding paradigm for the relationship between stress and illness, summarizing the background and development of the stress response:

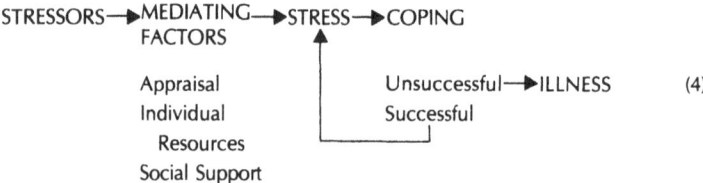

(4)

This concludes our introduction to current thinking and research into the nature of the stress response and its relationship to illness. Let us now go on to look at the impact stress can have upon general and specific aspects of illness.

LIFE EVENTS AND
ILLNESS

As mentioned in Chapter 1, the notion that significant life changes affect illness was first systematically explored by Adolph Meyer (Lief, 1948). In Chapters 1–4 we discussed how a stressor is defined and perceived by the individual, how it affects psychological and biological stress responses, and how individual and interpersonal factors can modify this response. Now we will focus on the impact all these factors together may have on health and illness, beginning with a review of the available evidence linking life stressors and illness.

THE MEASUREMENT OF LIFE EVENTS
AS THEY RELATE TO ILLNESS

The measurement of life events as stressors was greatly facilitated by the development of the Social Readjustment Rating Scale (SRRS) by Holmes and Rahe (1967). The SRRS is a standardized questionnaire of 43 stressing life events weighted according to psychophysical scaling methods. Each life event is given a mean value that represents the amount of adjustment the event would cause an individual in relation to his or her accustomed pattern of daily life. The amount of adjustment is based on an arbitrary value of 50 for marriage and adjustments for the remaining items are based on mean judgments taken from a sample of 394 subjects (see Table 3). The scaling of life events on this questionnaire has been reproduced by Ruch and Holmes (1971) with college students, and by Komaroff, Masuda, and Holmes (1968) with Black and Mexican Americans. In addition, there have been many cross-cultural replications validating the scaling of life events in the original Holmes and Rahe study. Masuda and Holmes (1967) compared Japanese and American samples; Harmon, Masuda, and Holmes (1970) collected American, Belgian, and Swiss samples; and Rahe (1969) compared American and Dutch populations with other groups. In general, these authors found that the stressor quality of these life events, in terms of their forcing changes in individual adjustment, is perceived in a remarkably similar fashion by a wide range of culturally diverse groups of people.

However, researchers have often modified the SRRS to meet specific needs of their own samples or to investigate particular kinds of stressors in particular kinds of situations. Wyatt (1977) reported that life-change events may be particularly affected by economic and social conditions among Black Americans and urged that attention be paid to how much such events contribute to overall life-stressor scores in different populations. Volicer, Isenberg, and Burns (1977) developed a separate measure, the Hospital Stress Rating Scale, to measure stress caused by hospitalization (see Table 4). Volicer (1978) reported that scores on this scale correlated positively with patients' reports of increased pain, lower physical status, and less improvement after discharge.

Modifying the scale is certainly justified when a researcher is concerned with a particular class of life stressors in a particular group of individuals, but in narrowing the focus, one runs the risk of losing the comparison with the extended body of literature available on the basic SRRS. However, one does gain the ability to specifically identify relevant stressors in the

TABLE 3. SOCIAL READJUSTMENT RATING SCALE

Rank	Life Event	Mean Value
1	Death of spouse	100
2	Divorce	73
3	Marital separation	65
4	Jail term	63
5	Death of close family member	63
6	Personal injury or illness	53
7	Marriage	50
8	Fired at work	47
9	Marital reconciliation	45
10	Retirement	45
11	Change in health of family member	44
12	Pregnancy	40
13	Sex difficulties	39
14	Gain of new family member	39
15	Business readjustment	39
16	Change in financial state	38
17	Death of close friend	37
18	Change to different line of work	36
19	Change in number of arguments with spouse	35
20	Mortgage over $10,000	31
21	Foreclosure of mortgage or loan	30
22	Change in responsibilities at work	29
23	Son or daughter leaving home	29
24	Trouble with in-laws	29
25	Outstanding personal achievement	28
26	Wife begin or stop work	26
27	Begin or end school	26
28	Change in living conditions	25
29	Revision of personal habits	24
30	Trouble with boss	23
31	Change in work hours or conditions	20
32	Change in residence	20
33	Change in schools	20
34	Change in recreation	19
35	Change in church activities	19
36	Change in social activities	18
37	Mortgage or loan less than $10,000	17
38	Change in sleeping habits	16
39	Change in number of family get-togethers	15
40	Change in eating habits	15
41	Vacation	13
42	Christmas	12
43	Minor violations of the law	11

(From Holmes and Rahe, 1967, Table 1, p. 214. Reprinted by permission of the *Journal of Psychosomatic Research*, Pergammon Press, Ltd.)

TABLE 4. HOSPITAL STRESS FACTORS

Factor	Stress Scale Events	Assigned Rank	Mean Rank Score
1. Unfamiliarity of surroundings	Having strangers sleep in the same room with you	01	13.9
	Having to sleep in a strange bed	03	15.9
	Having strange machines around	05	16.8
	Being awakened in the night by the nurse	06	16.9
	Being aware of unusual smells around you	11	19.4
	Being in a room that is too cold or too hot	16	21.7
	Having to eat cold or tasteless food	21	23.2
	Being cared for by an unfamiliar doctor	23	23.4
2. Loss of independence	Having to eat at different times than you usually do	02	15.4
	Having to wear a hospital gown	04	16.0
	Having to be assisted with bathing	07	17.0
	Not being able to get newspapers, radio or TV when you want them	08	17.7
	Having a roommate who has too many visitors	09	18.1
	Having to stay in bed or the same room all day	10	19.1
	Having to be assisted with a bedpan	13	21.5
	Not having your call light answered	35	27.3
	Being fed through tubes	39	29.2
	Thinking you may lose your sight	49	40.6
3. Separation from spouse	Worrying about your spouse being away from you	20	22.7
	Missing your spouse	38	28.4
4. Financial problems	Thinking about losing income because of your illness	27	25.9
	Not having enough insurance to pay for your hospitalization	36	27.4
5. Isolation from other people	Having a roommate who is seriously ill or cannot talk with you	12	21.2
	Having a roommate who is unfriendly	14	21.6
	Not having friends visit you	15	21.7
	Not being able to call family or friends on the phone	22	23.3
	Having the staff be in too much of a hurry	26	24.5
	Thinking you might lose your hearing	45	34.5
6. Lack of information	Thinking you might have pain because of surgery or test procedures	19	22.4
	Not knowing when to expect things will be done to you	25	24.2
	Having nurses or doctors talk too fast or use words you can't understand	29	26.4
	Not having your questions answered by the staff	37	27.6
	Not knowing the results or reasons for your treatments	41	31.9
	Not knowing for sure what illnesses you have	43	34.0
	Not being told what your diagnosis is	44	34.1
7. Threat of severe illness	Thinking your appearance might be changed after your hospitalization	17	22.1
	Being put in the hospital because of an accident	24	26.9
	Knowing you have to have an operation	32	26.9
	Having a sudden hospitalization you weren't planning to have	34	27.2
	Knowing you have a serious illness	46	34.6
	Thinking you might lose a kidney or some other organ	47	35.6
	Thinking you might have cancer	48	39.2
8. Separation from family	Being in the hospital during holidays or special family occasions	18	22.3
	Not having family visit you	31	26.5
	Being hospitalized far away from home	33	27.1
9. Problems with medications	Having medications cause you discomfort	28	26.0
	Feeling you are getting dependent on medications	30	26.4
	Not getting relief from pain medications	40	31.2
	Not getting pain medication when you need it	42	32.4

(From Volicer et al., 1977, Table 1, p. 7. Reprinted by permission of Opinion Publications, Inc., and the author.)

environment of interest. The general data supporting the SRRS provide a logical basis for constructing these types of specialized instruments.

The reliability of the SRRS as a life stressor measure has been supported by administering the same scale to the same subjects several different times. When Casey, Masuda, and Holmes (1967) retested a group of subjects after a nine-month waiting period, they found the subjects' evaluations of life-event stressors that had occurred during the past ten years to be remarkably stable. Thurlow (1971) reported the same stability for a two-week readministration of the scale covering life stressors during the past five years of the subjects' lives.

In general, SRRS research supports the crossed-sensitization hypothesis of the GAS following stressing events in human subjects. In a literature survey, Holmes and Masuda (1974) concluded "that life-change events . . . lower 'bodily resistance' and enhance the probability of disease occurrence." One potent measure of such indices would be the presence of physical distress following stressing events. Holmes and Holmes (1970) found the number of life-change events scored on the SRRS to be related to signs and symptoms of everyday life. Rahe, Mahan, and Arthur (1970) rank-ordered the crew of a naval vessel into four categories representing probability of illness according to SRRS scores and found a significant relationship between the rank-ordered categories and the illnesses that occurred while the ship was on cruise. Theorell and Rahe (1971) and Rahe and Paasikivi (1971) reported that SRRS scores for patients suffering heart attacks increased in the two years prior to their sickness. In addition, Thurlow (1971) found a significant correlation between yearly SRRS scores and consecutive periods of major illness.

The SRRS has also been used to study the relationship between life-stress events and symptoms of psychological distress. Using a modified version of the SRRS, Paykel et al. (1969) found a higher buildup of life-stress events in the six months prior to onset of depression in psychiatric hospital patients than in a matched control group. Uhlenhuth and Paykel (1973a) reported that symptom intensity in neurotic patients was significantly related to SRRS scores. In general, it has been reported that psychiatric patients exhibit higher SRRS scores than non-patients, although there are no significant differences between inpatients and outpatients (Uhlenhuth and Paykel, 1973b; Dekker and Webb, 1974). These elevated SRRS scores seem to correlate most highly with incidence of psychopathology when life stressors during the six months preceding the symptoms are measured (Paykel et al., 1969; Batlis, Webb, Dekker, and Muelheisen, 1972; Dekker and Webb, 1974; Bieliauskas and Webb, 1974).

The studies just mentioned demonstrate a retrospective relationship between SRRS scores and symptoms of distress, but the SRRS has also been shown to have some success in prospective prediction of illness in large human populations. Rahe, Mahan, and Arthur (1970) reported significant correlations between illness and SRRS scores for the most recent six-month period prior to cruise departure for 2600 Navy personnel on six- and eight-month cruises. Cline and Chosey (1972) found significant positive correlations between SRRS scores and the incidence of illness in a group of army cadets for predictive periods of two weeks, four months, eight months, and one year.

In general, this research has supported the notion that stressing life events are positively related to illness, thus apparently vindicating Adolph Meyer's early approach. However, as with all other stress-illness research, it has become apparent that stress-illness relationships are not nearly as straightforward as had been originally supposed.

Rubin, Gunderson, and Arthur (1971) administered the SRRS to crewmen on a Navy ship before a seven-month cruise and found that although subjects with high scores tended to have more illnesses, the differences were not significant. Aponte and Miller (1972), using the SRRS in a psychiatric population, found a relationship between life-stress events and the patient's past psychiatric history, but little relationship between life-stress events and the patient's present psychiatric status.

Bieliauskas and Webb (1974) further questioned the significant relationships demonstrated by the SRRS between life-stress events and symptoms of physical or psychological maladjustment. Their study found that a significant relationship existed between the incidence of stressing events and the incidence of aid-seeking in college students—generally confirming the relationship between life stressors and illness found in other studies. However their statistical analysis of the amount of aid-seeking that could be accounted for by life-stress suggested that it was quite small. In comparing their study and other studies, the amount of illness that can be accounted for by life stressors could not be computed above 5 percent. Wershow and Reinhart (1974, p. 400) reported that although SRRS scores increased in the months prior to hospitalization for eighty-eight male patients, this "may be statistically significant, but is obviously of little clinical significance. . . . The point has been amply made that some relationship exists between change in life-ways, let alone stress, and illness. However, the relationship is a weak one." Caplan (1975) suggested that one reason for this lack of a strong, albeit significant, relationship between life-stress events and illness may be that these events do not have the same importance for each individual.

The notion of striking differences between individual reactions to stressors has been emphasized throughout this volume. Most of the studies of general life-event relationships with illness have been done with large groups. Although this approach may well uncover life events that are stressors for most people (such as divorce or death of a spouse), it neglects all those individual aspects we discussed earlier – cognitive appraisal, social mediators, actual stress, and coping. Thus, the issue of how life stressors affect illness in individual cases continues to be unresolved. Bieliauskas and Strugar (1976) demonstrated that relationships between life-stress measurement and aid-seeking become steadily less robust as the size of the group being examined decreased. Nevertheless, it is well worth reviewing the attempts that have been made to identify important parameters in measurement of life-stress events and their impact on health and illness.

INDEPENDENCE OF LIFE EVENTS FROM ILLNESS

Dohrenwend (1974) raised the point that a number of the life events listed in the SRRS may actually be part of the illness process itself. For example, an event such as change in sexual functioning may well be the *result* of an individual's illness, such as flu, rather than a predecessor to it. If life stressors are measured during the course of an illness, it may be difficult to tell whether the changes came before the illness or after its onset. Hudgens (1974) suggests that 29 of the life events on the SRRS may fall into this category. Dohrenwend and Dohrenwend (1978, p. 9) suggested that "this kind of bias in a sample of life events seriously limits the kinds of inferences that can be drawn from a correlation between the number or magnitude of events experienced and illness." The basic problem becomes one of interpreting causality. Large studies have rarely taken such distinctions into account and their findings may well have been prejudiced towards showing larger-than-life relationships between life events and illness. On a more individual level, however, careful and detailed inquiry may possibly help us uncover the actual relationship between life stressors and illness.

DESIRABLE LIFE EVENTS

As can be seen in Table 3, not all the life changes listed are necessarily aversive; for example, taking a vacation might be a welcome break from routine chores. Initially, this was not felt to be significant because all the events were chosen for the degree of adjustment they required rather than for their pleasant or unpleasant characteristics. However, Gersten, Langner, Eisenberg, and Orzek (1974), in a study of delinquency and general intellectual functioning in a sample of children and young adults, found that the desirability of a life event *did* have significant impact on how events relate to various outcomes. Selye (1974) also noted that good stressors led to effective adjustment and bad stressors led to poor adjustment. However, this distinction seems to be more related to the way each individual reacted to environmental events rather than to the characteristics of the events themselves. Lazarus et al. (1980) elaborated on this notion and found that different individuals are likely to see the same event as good or bad depending on the context and effects of a given stressor. Thus, the distinction between pleasant and unpleasant events, in and of themselves, may be neither significant nor possible to make.

The important questions are whether or not the appearance of a stressor is (1) perceived as a stressor, and (2) coped with successfully. If a stressor is not coped with effectively, then it will probably continue to evoke a stress response, possibly leading to eventual illness. Thus, it might be more useful to view events as causing or not causing continued stress rather than as being good or bad.

PREDICTABILITY AND CONTROL OF LIFE EVENTS

In Chapter 3 we discussed the importance of being able to

predict the occurrence of a stressor and to control it (to cope with it). In general terms, the research has suggested that a lack of predictability or control increases stress, although not under all circumstances. Dohrenwend and Dohrenwend (1978) confirmed that the ability to anticipate and control the occurence of a noxious stimulus tends to ameliorate its effects. They cite the work of Glass, Singer, and Friedman (1969) as a demonstration of this interaction. In that study, a predictable noise produced less disruption of a proofreading task than did random noise, and subjects performed better on a similar task if they were told they could turn off the noise if it became unbearable.

The implications of predictability and control of stressors for health and illness were discussed in Chapter 3, where "giving up" was noted as a precursor of eventual illness. The individual's perception of his ability to cope with a stressor thus has an effect on the stress response and on subsequent illness. For example, it is well known that patients who are well prepared for medical procedures tend to have a better recovery. Prenatal classes on the events of childbirth can ease deliveries by providing realistic information about anticipated pain, physiological changes, and technical procedures, and by giving the mother-to-be some means of coping with unpleasant sensations through relaxation techniques such as those used in the Lamaze method of childbirth (Bing, 1969). Klein et al. (1968) provided evidence that advance preparation may also be important in recovery from heart attack. They studied heart patients who were transferred from intensive care units, and found that adverse emotional and physical consequences resulted from the patients' inability to predict or control changes in their environments.

Thus, if medical procedures are stressors, patients' stress responses can be minimized if they are given a clear explanation of what will probably happen (prediction) and close consultation about the options that are available (control) to them. Less stress should in turn produce faster recovery and better physical stability. From my own consultations with hospitalized patients, I can attest on the one hand to the emotional upset caused by having unexpected procedures (such as an EKG monitor) applied when the patient has no idea of the necessity or purpose of the procedure. On the other hand, I have also seen patients willingly give multiple blood samples once they were made aware of the intervals between the samples and the reason the procedure had been ordered (such as monitoring drug dosage levels).

Again, these issues have not been fully addressed in life-event research, partially because the SRRS and similar instruments of measurement are insensitive to them, and partially because delineation of such parameters is extremely difficult in large group studies. Again, on an individual, clinical level, careful inquiry and consultation with patients may well provide pertinent information about how predictability and control affect patient reactions to stressors such as medical procedures. It is generally accepted that these two factors have a significant effect on the nature of the stress response.

ILLNESS VERSUS ILLNESS BEHAVIOR

When life-event and illness relationships are being investigated, it is important to determine whether it is actual illness or illness behavior that is being measured. *Illness* is the subjective phenomenon of being sick, and it may be manifested by physical symptoms and signs of disease or by a general sense of malaise for which there is no discernible physical basis. *Illness behavior,* on the other hand, refers to how the individual responds once the subjective perception of illness has been made. The response may involve staying home from work, easing away from responsibilities, or seeking medical advice. White, Williams, and Greenberg (1961) noted that only about one-third of the people who reported symptoms serious enough to require medical care actually sought it out. Mechanic (1976) more specifically reported that despite the general frequency of symptoms of viral respiratory disease in the population, only a small number of such cases are brought to the attention of a physician. Mechanic (1976) suggested that rather than influencing illness, stress may actually influence illness behavior, since it is the factor of seeking medical care that generally comes to the attention of the researcher. Tessler, Mechanic, and Dimond (1976) suggested that subjective distress like the discomfort associated with a variety of personal and extrapersonal conflicts plays a large role in determining whether medical help is sought out, even when sociodemographic, attributional, and health status factors are controlled. Mechanic (1978, p. 30) concluded that the "level of distress is the single most important predictor of help-seeking." In this sense, stressors seem to primarily affect attempts to cope with illness (by seeking medical help) rather than the illness itself. This distinction has not always been made in research addressing relationships between stress and illness.

Because the diagnosis of illness by medical personnel must, by definition, be the result of illness behavior (the patient's having come to a medical facility), distinguishing between the illness and its related behaviors is quite difficult under any circumstances. It has proven extremely difficult to obtain reliable subjective descriptions of illness from groups of subjects not seeking medical care. The data resulting from questionnaires that have been used for such studies have been generally impossible to verify. However, the distinction between illness and illness behavior may be crucial to understanding stress-illness relationships for two main reasons. First, illness behavior is a way of coping with a stressor, and thus would be expected to be related to stress, either as a direct method of coping with the stress of being ill or as a means of coping with an illness resulting from a prolonged stress response. Moreover, seeking help may be activated by the presence of life stressors when mild illness symptoms exist; if the stressors were not present, the same illness symptoms might not lead the patient to seek medical attention. Thus, it may be impossible to make a distinction between the two, since the stressors may be having an effect on both illness and illness behavior simultaneously. Second, if we think that stress-illness relationships provide us with clues for developing effective intervention strategies to promote health, illness behavior is the point at which some action must be taken. We can do little about curing or preventing illness if we never know it exists.

Our inability to make a distinction between illness and illness behavior does not necessarily impugn the utility of the stress-illness perspective, even though it may blur the divisions in our paradigm of stress and illness, such as coping versus the end-point of illness. On a research level, this general distinction remains a challenge, but on the clinical level it may well be enough to be able to make some distinctions when dealing with an individual patient who can provide us with a thorough history of life stressors, illness symptoms, signs, and coping strategies.

PAST HISTORY OF ILLNESS AND THRESHOLD EFFECT FOR STRESSORS

Although the term "stressor" can be applied to large classes of life events based on general, cross-cultural data, we also know that even under the worst circumstances, such as war or natural catastrophe, some individuals become ill and others do not. Most studies showing relationships between illness and research instruments like the SRRS use subjects from physically or psychiatrically pathological groups. In studies based on "healthy" subjects (such as the ones conducted by Holmes and Masuda, 1974), groups of subjects who became ill had higher life-change scores than groups who remained healthy. However, we have no information on whether there were significantly high life-change scores among the subjects in these groups who did *not* become ill. There are always a number of individuals in "not-ill" comparison groups who have high life-change scores even though the overall scores for the "not-ill" group are lower than the overall scores of the "ill" group. A series of studies by Hinkle (1974) may help shed some light on this question. In long-term studies of telephone workers, Hinkle found that stressing life events apparently precipitated illness only in those individuals with pre-existing patterns of illness; that is, in those subjects who might be said to be "predisposed" to illness. Even stressors of large magnitude did not precipitate illness in those subjects who were *not* predisposed to illness. Garrity, Marx, and Somes (1977) further reported that "correlations between life change and health change [in college students] generally increased over the study period, especially with outcomes indicative of more severe illness." Holmes and Masuda (1974) suggest that the role played by changing life events in precipitating illness may be that of a necessary, although not sufficient, cause. Thus, knowing whether or not an individual has a past history of becoming ill may help us predict whether that individual will develop illness in the face of future life stressors.

Another parameter that may affect the relationship between stress and illness was suggested by Bieliauskas and Strugar (1976). They found the SRRS to have varying success at predicting which college students would seek aid. Seeking aid appeared to be related to overall levels of SRRS scores; the higher the general scores for all subjects tested, the more likely it was that higher and lower scores within the sample could differentiate those who would seek aid for medical or psychological reasons from those who would not. Bieliauskas and Strugar also found indications that life-event scores will discriminate aid-seekers from non-aid-seekers only in populations that generally experience an increased number of life events. Wildman and Johnson (1977) described this as the "threshold effect" of life change; that is, there is a finite amount of life stress that has to occur before an individual will notice deleterious effects taking place. A number of other investigators have supported this finding (Theorell, 1976; Crandall and Lehman, 1977; Wildman, 1978).

In a study that looked at the incidence of life-stressing events, stress response as measured by 17-OHCS levels, and aid-seeking, Bieliauskas (1980) was unable to demonstrate significant relationships between any of these variables. However, the subjects studied were all employed, relatively healthy firefighters who had little history of illness, at least illness serious enough to require hospitalization or to prevent working. Although these results may not seem to support the stress-illness hypotheses, the variables of past illness history and the threshold effect may have played an important part in the failure to demonstrate significant relationships. Based on the results of this study as compared with those previously mentioned in this chapter, Bieliauskas (1980) suggested that perhaps a relationship between stress and illness may only be demonstrable when the factors of current general stress level and history of past illness are elevated. The interactive model proposed can be seen in Figure 11.

INDIVIDUAL IMPACT OF LIFE-STRESSING EVENTS

By definition the SRRS is a group measure of the average amount of life adjustment experienced by individuals in

Maladjustment History

		Hi	Lo
Stress Level	Hi	High Relationship	Intermediate Relationship
	Lo	Intermediate Relationship	Low Relationship

FIGURE 11. Model for degree of relationship between stressing life events and maladjustment. (From Bieliauskas, 1980, Figure 2, p. 34. Reprinted by permission of Opinion Publications, Inc., and the author.)

response to particular life stressors. However, as we have pointed out, each individual experiences different life events in different ways. Redfield and Stone (1979) demonstrated that if the SRRS was given to a group of individuals who rated the individual items along several dimensions, the individuals rated different qualities of the items in different ways. Furthermore, the difference in how individuals rated life events appeared to be related to how much adjustment each life event seemed to entail. The earlier work done on the reliability of the SRRS dealt with generally similar rankings of items across wide groups of subjects, but in a more detailed analysis of item rankings, Volicer (1978) demonstrated that on a scale of life stressors related to hospitalization, life-event items that required larger adjustments tended to be ranked similarly, while there was no consensus in the ranking of events that required a lesser adjustment. The implication here is that in any life scale, particularly stressing life events will tend to be seen similarly, while less stressing events will be ranked in a variety of ways.

Attempts have been made to develop scales to measure individually experienced stressing effects of different life events. Horowitz, Wilner, and Alvarez (1979) developed such a scale, but it was related to a specific theory of stress response (see Chapter 7), and its application to general stress-illness considerations is unclear. Reeder, Scharama, and Dirken (1973) developed a Subjective Stress Scale designed to measure individual reactions to stressors. Croog and Fitzgerald (1978) used this scale to measure the impact of life stressors on wives of men who had experienced first-time heart attacks. They found that although scores on the Subjective Stress Scale were significantly related to generally stressing life experiences, to unhappiness, and to emotional vulnerability, they were not significantly related to symptoms of illness. Croog and Fitzgerald's study was conducted over a relatively short period (one year) so the implications of their findings for the long-term effects of stress on illness are unclear. However, the results do suggest that increasing unhappiness and emotional vulnerability may be related to seeking medical help. Continued research with such scales will be necesssary to evaluate the significance of their contribution to the understanding of stress-illness relationships.

SCALES OF COMBINED CHARACTERISTICS OF LIFE EVENTS

Given the criticisms of measuring stressing life-events in a general fashion, several attempts have been made to develop more discriminating scales. Ruch (1977) employed the SRRS in an attempt to measure different aspects of how subjects rated items on the scale. Each subject was asked first to rate SRRS items according to the original directions used by Holmes and Rahe (1967) and then to rate each item with specific attention to the amount of adaptation required and the time that adaptation would take. Their ratings were subjected to an analysis that grouped the rated items along statistical dimensions. Three main dimensions emerged from that analysis: (1) the degree of life change required, (2) the desirability of the life change, and (3) the area of the life change (work versus home, for example). Thus, it is clear that an instrument like the SRRS is also subject to the influence of some of the characteristics we have been discussing. Dohrenwend, Krasnoff, Askenasy, and Dohrenwend (1978) have made probably the most elegant attempt yet to design a scale that takes many of these characteristics into account—the Psychiatric Epidemiology Research Interview Life Events Scale (PERI). The researchers gathered life events in a community by asking a large number of people from differing ethnic and socioeconomic backgrounds which recent events in their lives were most stressing. The scale was designed to control for specific versus general stress effects (that is, whether the life event was important only for a particular individual or group or for a broader range of the population), for the desirability or undesirability of the life events, for the dependence or independence of the life event from an illness process, and for the individual's ability to control the occurrence of the life event. The PERI is only now beginning to be used to further investigate stress-illness relationships, but is clearly a step in the right direction, moving us closer to a full consideration of the many factors affecting such relationships.

DO STRESSING LIFE EVENTS AFFECT ILLNESS?

General evidence on the relationship between stressing life events and illness suggests that there *is* a positive relationship, although the evidence is certainly not overwhelming. We now know that a wide range of individual factors must be taken into account when investigating stress, factors that have often not been considered in stress-illness studies. It is also true that a number of parameters specifically important to life-events research are often not included in larger group studies. These parameters include the independence of life events from illness, the desirability of life events, the predictability and control of life events, the measurement of illness versus illness behavior, the past history of illness, possible threshold effects for life stress, and the individual impact of life events.

The task of assessing the impact of stressors on illness for individual patients is exceedingly complex, as our discussion has shown. However, there are guidelines we can follow in determining the vulnerability of an individual to illness once we know what that person perceives as a stressor. Does the patient have enough personal and interpersonal resources to cope with the stressor? Has he or she had success coping with such stressors in the past? Does the patient feel some degree of confidence in his ability to predict and cope with the stressor? Is the stressor a byproduct of the illness? Is there a past history of general health? Is the patient free of other general stressors? The research we have reviewed suggests that negative answers to these questions increase the probability that stressing life events will lead to illness for that person.

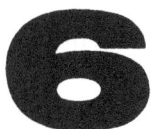

PSYCHOPHYSIOLOGICAL
REACTIONS TO STRESS

Now that we have discussed the psychological and biological background of stress and how stress is generally related to illness, let us consider the specific kinds of illnesses that stress has been linked to and look at how the linkage may affect treatment. In this chapter, we will concentrate on illnesses classified as "psychophysiological." A psychophysiological disorder is one "in which organ and visceral symptomatology is produced by emotional factors acting through the autonomic nervous system" (Kolb, 1973). We will not dwell on the relationship between specific end-organ problems and the autonomic nervous system as the result of exposure to stress because, as noted in Chapter 1, if a given individual has had previous dysfunction in a particular organ system, he is then generally predisposed to have recurring dysfunction in that system when exposed to stress. (A good text on medical physiology can provide details about the functioning of the autonomic nervous system if you wish to look into the matter more fully.) We will continue to explore the general effects of stress, focusing now on specific symptoms.

HEADACHES

The most common types of headaches generally encountered are either vascular in nature (such as migraines) or caused by contractions (such as tension headaches). Both types of headaches are commonly associated with hyperalertness, work pressures, frustration, and an excessive output of energy. They often occur in conjunction with feelings of anger or resentment (Wolf and Goodell, 1968) and are commonly regarded as indicative of stressors in the environment. The source of pain in vascular headaches seems to be the vasoconstriction or dilation of intracranial and extracranial arteries, while in tension headaches, the source of pain is thought to be "sustained contraction of muscles in the forehead, scalp, and neck" (Pomerleau, 1979). Marcussen and Wolff (1949) showed clearly that headaches can be a reaction to psychological stressors. They were able to bring on headaches in their subjects by the use of "stress-inducing" interview techniques that involved discussing personal topics in a way that created resentment and guilt. The stressors most commonly associated with headaches are psychological in nature; we frequently get headaches when faced with stressors that severely tax our ability to cope, such as job pressures, extended periods of fatigue, and interpersonal strife—thus the often-heard phrase, "That gives me a headache." Williams (1977, p. 43) described the etiology of such headaches as follows:

> The tension level in the muscles of the head and neck has been shown to increase in experimental studies in response to a wide variety of psychological as well as physical stimuli—and as little as two minutes of sustained voluntary contraction is associated with the onset of pain in the contracting muscles. Other experimental studies have shown that the arteries of the scalp constrict in response to unpleasant physical and psychological stimuli. Persons with a high need to be in control—who maintain that control by meticulously ordering their environment—are going to be subjected frequently to frustration of that need. The

result of such frustration is then likely to be preparation for an emergency response with the result that the muscles of the head and neck contract, the blood vessels of the scalp constrict, and with enough frustration, over a sufficient length of time, a headache develops.

As you may realize by now, we can intervene in the headache's development stress model, anywhere from removing or changing the perception of a stressor to actually treating the illness itself. Treatment of stress-related headache is what Lazarus (1977) described as direct management of somatic turmoil; that is, treatment of the end-organ response to stress.

Treating headaches involves finding ways to relax the vasospasms and muscle tension associated with onset. Of all the treatment approaches for relaxing muscular tension, electromyographic (EMG) feedback has received the most attention. In this approach a monitor attached to the patient measures muscle tension (usually in the frontalis muscle of the forehead) and sounds an audible tone the patient can hear. If tension increases, the tone also increases in pitch or in loudness; it decreases when tension also decreases. The patient can thus directly monitor his muscle tension levels and work at modifying them. Budzynski (1977) reported that although EMG feedback is generally successful in easing the effects of headaches, it may not be the agent directly responsible for the change. Haynes, Griffin, Mooney, and Parise (1975) suggested that teaching a patient general passive relaxation techniques could reduce tension headaches as well as EMG feedback. Silver and Blanchard (1978), in a review of the literature, found that relaxation training alone was as effective as EMG biofeedback. Cohen, McArthur, and Rickles (1980) found no difference between different types of biofeedback treatment. The EMG biofeedback approach may well help reduce the stress response (and thereby, the headache) by generally strengthening coping skills, rather than by specifically reducing the headache. However, this issue is complex and has not yet been resolved (Belar, 1978).

In addition to EMG biofeedback for muscular tension, migraine headaches have often been treated with similar biofeedback techniques that monitor temperature changes in the fingers. A monitor is attached to the patient's fingers and temperature changes are transformed into an audible signal the patient can hear. The patient is then instructed to warm his hands, the theory being that this will increase peripheral circulation and thus divert blood flow from painfully distended cranial arteries. The effectiveness of this approach is highly speculative. In a recent article, Lake, Rainey, and Papsdorf (1979) reported that EMG feedback procedures were generally more effective than temperature feedback in decreasing migraine headache and questioned the effectiveness of the temperature approach. Dalessio (1972) suggested that the important factor in changing migraine headache frequency was changing the patient's general cognitive appraisal of stressors. Both Lake et al. (1979) and Budzynski (1977) found that home practice of EMG techniques was a crucial factor in reducing headaches. This may indicate that a general change in coping with stressors is at work rather than a specific headache reduction effect.

Thus, the basic effectiveness of biofeedback techniques, especially EMG feedback, is pretty much accepted although we do not yet know whether the techniques themselves are what eliminate the symptoms. It may be that the techniques mainly aid the patient by helping him develop a broader range of coping responses.

BACK PAIN

Pain is a subjective phenomenon that is difficult to quantify.

There are no known direct physical measurements that can reflect the amount of pain a patient is experiencing or tell us when the pain has been effectively relieved by treatment. All we have to go on is the patient's own report.

Quite a bit of research has been done to try and quantify patients' reports of pain. Some early work on developing a questionnaire to categorize descriptors of pain was carried out by Melzack and Torgerson (1971). They classified a number of words describing pain along factorial dimensions. Their technique was later refined by Leavitt, Garron, Whisler, and Sheinkop (1978) into a back-pain scale that seemed able to account for significant proportions of lower-back-pain experiences. This scale allowed patients to describe affective (emotionally-related) as well as sensory (detection-related) dimensions of back pain.

In 1979, Leavitt, Garron, and Bieliauskas used a scale developed by Leavitt et al. (1978) to evaluate relationships between pain and life stressors. They found that life stressors were significantly related to affective pain dimensions, but not to other dimensions. This was true only if organic contributors to the pain could not be identified. In 1980, Leavitt, Garron, and Bieliauskas found that life-stressing events were elevated in patients with psychometrically verified psychological disturbances, but not in others. In this case, the existence of organic contributors to pain did not seem to make a difference; patients with and without demonstrated organic injury showed elevated experience of life events if psychological disturbance could be documented.

The results of these studies suggest that the mere occurrence of stressing life events does not in and of itself predispose a person to lower back pain. Nor do the results support assertions that back-pain symptoms are a somatic reaction to stress per se (Fordyce, 1976; Wooley, Blackwell, and Winget, 1978). However, the Leavitt et al. studies do indicate that there is some relationship between life-stressing events and psychological disturbance in lower-back-pain patients. This is consistent with the notion that there is a subgroup of patients with lower back pain who have a disturbed ability to cope with stressors and that in this subgroup affective (emotionally distressing) aspects of pain may be exacerbated by life stress.

Attempts at modification of chronic pain of any kind, including back pain, have been attempted, but not with as well-documented success as other researchers have had with headaches (Gentry and Bernal, 1977). Such approaches also use EMG biofeedback techniques, again, usually with frontalis muscle tension, in an attempt to teach patients to generally relax tension throughout the body. Sternbach (1974) and Fordyce (1976) emphasize the need for a more general approach than this, one that would teach patients different ways of interacting with their environments in order to eliminate behaviors contributing to pain and to provide patients with more general coping mechanisms for dealing with stressors.

The research of Leavitt et al., Sternbach, and Fordyce supports the claim that intervention through teaching patients how to cope effectively with stress is a sound approach. We have seen how a general failure to cope with stressors brings on an increased stress response and subsequent somatic symptoms. Clearly, the work of modifying pain in this way is in its infancy, but the stress paradigm we have followed throughout this volume appears to be relevant and will surely be part of future studies.

ASTHMA

Asthma is generally defined as a tendency toward bronchoconstriction that impedes respiration. Wolf and Goodell (1968) have described studies involving subjects who historically reacted to stressors with allergic asthmatic attacks. These individuals developed asthma when subjected to nonspecific physical stressors (such as the tightening of a fitted steel crown about their heads) or to psychological stressors (such as the mention of personal conflicts). Wolf and Goodell believe that asthma can also be experimentally induced in susceptible individuals (those with a history of asthma) by emotionally troublesome events. Weiner (1977) also noted that in clinical observation, asthma attacks are frequently preceded by emotional tension, but he questioned the assumption of a cause-effect relationship. Asthma usually develops in childhood, and the effect of this handicap on the development of appropriate emotional responses to daily conflicts may be more important than the effect of the stressors on the illness.

Alexander (1977, p. 15) listed three basic approaches used in the treatment of asthma: one can try "(1) to alter the abnormal pulmonary functioning more or less directly; (2) to alter maladaptive emotional concomitants; and (3) to alter maladaptive asthma-related behaviors and family patterns. . . . The methods which are intended to alter lung function in asthma include relaxation training, biofeedback, direct operant conditioning, and to some extent the deconditioning methods." In addition to the general and specific techniques we have already discussed, the conditioning methods Alexander referred to are psychologically applied attempts to "unlearn" asthma as a coping response. Alexander noted some success with these approaches, but he stressed that a combination of medical and behavior methods was usually most effective. The same point was made by Hock, Rodgers, Reddi, and Kennard (1978), who found that relaxation techniques were quite effective in increasing respiratory functioning and decreasing the frequency of asthma attacks, while changing general behavioral coping patterns alone had little effect. Kinsman, Dirks, Jones, and Dahlem (1980), however, caution against using relaxation techniques alone, arguing that they may not be appropriate in many cases. Again, a combination of medical and behavioral approaches appears to be called for.

Asthma is thus a complex illness that appears to require direct medical intervention although it may also respond to interventions based on modifying coping techniques focused on end-organ responses (learning not to react with asthma in stressing situations) or on general relaxation. Again, our model of the stress response process fits the research findings. Individuals with a history of asthma seem to have recurring symptoms in the face of stressors, even though the actual symptom complex may well be due to physical factors. Modifying either the response itself or the coping abilities used to deal with stressors (thus reducing the stress response) appear to be effective approaches to intervention in this illness.

ULCERATION IN THE VISCERA

In 1968, Wolf and Goodell conducted studies that showed that gastric hyperfunctioning leads to erosions of the stomach and intestinal wall, with increases in hydrochloric acid activity. The Brady (1958) and Weiss (1970, 1972) studies cited earlier clearly related the onset of stressors and certain methods of coping to visceral lesions. Ulceration is also one of the "diseases of adaptation" described by Selye (1956). This idea is somewhat supported by the fact that patients undergoing corticosteroid therapy commonly run the risk of ulcerations of the stomach, as do those with Cushing's Disease (hyperfunctioning of the adrenal gland). There is also an element of constitutional predisposition; ulceration seems to run in families, and Weiner (1977) found evidence that ulcer patients have common psychological characteristics, especially a need to be loved and cared for and significant conflicts over independence versus dependence. Weiner also reviewed studies in which gastric secretion increased in subjects who were experiencing personal conflict or anxiety. The increased secretions have lasted as long as several days when the psychological pressures persisted.

Ulcers are commonly recognized as a hazard of working in high-pressure environments. As with headaches, a common popular saying, "I'm going to get an ulcer from this," may accurately reflect the stress-related nature of work or emotional pressures. However, the evidence on how ulcers are caused is not entirely clear. Selye felt that ulcers might be a crossed-sensitization response; that is, the protective lining of the stomach can be seen as an inflammatory response that prevents erosion of the mucosal wall until adaptation to stress causes anti-inflammatory changes in the lining. This is purely speculative, however. The evidence for increased acid secretion in individuals experiencing conflict is not entirely explanatory; in one study (Fordtran, 1973), only one-third to one-half of the peptic ulcer patients secreted excessive amounts of gastric acid. What could be causing the ulcers of the remaining patients?

The connection between stress and ulceration of the viscera is thus ambiguous; it is a theoretically attractive idea, yet it is far from having been conclusively demonstrated. Treatments for peptic ulcers range from recommendations to "take a vacation" or "change jobs" to drug and surgical therapies. The former are clearly related to coping with stressors and modifying the stress response, while the latter are focused on modifying the end-organ response. Generally, both types of approaches are used, if possible. It is thus likely that future treatment approaches will be related to our stress-illness paradigm, although at this point the evidence is not overwhelming.

HEART DISEASE

Dysfunctions of the heart musculature can be related to

malfunctions of the autonomic nervous system and to other factors, such as serum cholesterol levels, smoking, and alcohol consumption. However, since the actions of the nervous system in cardial regulation are primarily involuntary, we will focus on general heart disease in this chapter. We will start by describing the relationships between the popular concept of the "Type A Personality" and heart disease from a stress-illness viewpoint and then we will look at evidence directly relating stress to various cardiac dysfunctions.

The Type A Personality

Friedman and Rosenman (1974) felt that the general increase in heart disease during the last fifty years was related to the stresses and challenges of our increasingly complex civilization. This increasing complexity has given rise to a set of behaviors they termed the "Type A coronary-prone behavior pattern." This behavior pattern is "an action-emotion complex that can be observed in any person who is aggressively involved in a chronic, incessant struggle to achieve more and more in less and less time, and, if required, to do so against the opposing effects of other things or persons." These behaviors are more specifically described by Glass (1977) as "competitive achievement striving, a sense of time urgency, and hostility." In general, Glass suggests that Type A individuals are extremely threatened by a loss of control over environmental events and are therefore constantly striving to maintain control. Research cited by Glass suggests that Type A individuals tend to work close to their ultimate levels of endurance on all tasks, even on easy ones that do not require such expenditure of effort. However, when faced with an uncontrollable task, Type A individuals tend to "give up" more easily than others, hypothetically because they cannot accept the possibility of losing control.

Many of the themes of Type A behavior should already be

familiar to you from our earlier discussions. We have explored the interactions between past illness, predictability, and the control of stressors, as well as how helplessness in the face of threat is a good indication of a poor outcome. In addition, there is now evidence that Type A behaviors are related to changes in catecholamine secretion (Rosenman and Friedman, 1974) and serum lipids (Suinn, Brock, and Edie, 1975), the hormonal factors in the stress response that we discussed in Chapter 2. The application of our stress-illness paradigm to Type A behavior appears to be quite direct. Glass (1977) pointed out that Type A behavior is not an all-pervasive factor; rather it appears in the face of stressors that threaten the patient's control. Thus, Type A behavior can be viewed as a way of coping with stress. One of the costs of such an adaptation, however, appears to be heart disease.

The general nature of Type A behavior may also be familiar to you in a personal sense. Individuals in health-related professions are frequently educated in programs that almost demand such behavior, and the work environment frequently does the same. The irony of this situation, if you look around you, is that those individuals who exhibit Type A behaviors are frequently more successful than those who do not. Therefore, the environmental situation is geared to reward such behaviors and thus perpetuates them.

What is the actual risk of Type A behavior for heart disease? In an eight-year follow-up of individuals initially identified as Type A's, Rosenman et al. (1975) found that Type A's had more than twice the rate of heart disease as individuals who did not exhibit the Type A behavior pattern. This was true even when conventional risk indicators were controlled (Orth-Gomer, Ahlborn, and Theorell, 1980). In addition, socially insecure Type A's tended to have more serious instances of atherosclerosis (Jenkins et al., 1977), and Type A's in general showed greater increases in blood pressure in response to stressing interviews than individuals who did not evidence Type A behaviors (Dembroski, MacDougall, and Lushene, 1979). The likelihood of Type A individuals developing heart disease or other risk factors associated with coronary disease appears to be considerable.

What can be done about the risks of Type A behavior? Before we can intervene, we must be able to identify the pattern. The Jenkins Activity Survey for Health Prediction (Jenkins, Zyzanski, and Rosenman, 1979) is a self-administered questionnaire that can be scored to evaluate whether that individual is classifiable as Type A. Glass (1977) has suggested that the basic intervention required for Type A individuals is a major change in coping style. Attempts to accomplish such changes have included the administration of sedative psychotropic drugs (Sigg, 1974), Transcendental Meditation (Benson, Marzetta, and Rosner, 1974), general relaxation and tension-reduction approaches (Roskies et al., 1978; Cooper and Aygen, 1979), and excercise (Blumenthal, Williams, Williams, and Wallace, 1980). All of these techniques have been shown to effectively reduce cardiac risk factors at the time of treatment, but only a few studies have made extended follow-up investigations to see if the initial improvements were maintained (Roskies et al., 1979). Some authors like, Friedman and Rosenman (1977), even believe that it is futile to attempt to change Type A behaviors until an actual heart attack has occurred. Given the fact that Type A behaviors develop over long periods and are often strongly reinforced, it is not surprising that patients are reluctant to change their ways. Type A behavior modification is still in an early stage of development and its long-term efficacy has not yet been proved.

General Cardiac Risk Factors

Hypertension. High blood pressure can be affected by a

wide spectrum of stimuli related to stressing life experiences, from one-time single stressors to ongoing daily pressures. Wolf and Goodell (1968) have pointed out that blood pressure changes are only significant to potential heart disease when they are profound and sustained over time. Weiner (1977) has also attested to the manipulability of blood pressure in experimental situations.

There are many risk factors for hypertension—smoking, alcohol consumption, age, and race, to name a few. As you might suspect, isolating the influence of specific stressors from this array of contributors is quite difficult. Nevertheless, it is now clear that in the laboratory situation, blood pressure can be manipulated through feedback techniques, although the mechanics of manipulation in terms of rate, time, systole versus diastole, and so on are quite complex (Schwartz, 1977). There is no real evidence that experimental manipulation of hypertension has any lasting effects. In a critical review of this issue, Shekelle (1979, p. 1249) found this lack of evidence compelling: "Hypertension has not been shown to bear a consistent relationship with psychological attributes—anxiety, suppressed hostility, and neuroticism, for instance—or with exposure to stressful situations, such as rapid sociocultural change." However, Shekelle did feel that when stress could be linked to various coping behaviors considered to have significant impact on cardiac risk factors (such as smoking and drinking) attempts to manage stress might be quite productive. It is not uncommon for behavioral interventions in the management of blood pressure to have some overt or covert effects on such risk factors, and the distinction between the type of effects may be quite difficult to make.

At present, the relationship between stress and hypertension is unproven. Whether it is the complexity of the interaction that makes this relationship difficult to discover or whether no relationship exists remains to be seen.

Arrhythmias. Ursin et al. (1978), whose work was described in Chapter 2, also found accelerated heart rates in their parachute jumping trainees during each attempted jump. They interpreted this tachycardia as being related to increased psychological activation, since it could not be correlated with increased oxygen intake. Interestingly, unlike the hormonal measures, heart rate did not change over time (with coping) but remained stable throughout the training period. Blix, Stromme, and Ursin (1974) noted a similar increase in heart rate in pilots at the time of landing and takeoff, even when they had had considerable experience in the air. It appears that heart-rate acceleration occurs when the nature and time of the stressor are uncertain; deceleration occurs when the stressor is familiar and occurs predictably (Ursin et al., 1978). Natelson and Cagin (1979) have also reported the occurrence of ventricular arrhythmias in response to stressors.

The combined findings of these studies point to stressors and various aspects of the stressor/stress/coping interaction as central to the activation of irregular heart rates. However, these irregularities would only cause illness if they continued over extended periods. There is no evidence that such prolonged changes occur with any regularity nor that they are directly related to stress. Biofeedback techniques have also been successful in regulating heart rate (Schwartz, 1977), although again, no one has done follow-up studies to see if the positive effects are continued over time.

Whether induced changes in heart rate are strongly connected to subsequent heart disease is highly questionable. They are probably a byproduct of other activated processes rather than a pathological effect in and of themselves.

CONCLUSIONS

The importance of stress in psychophysiological illness has

been supported by the evidence on both a theoretical and a tangible basis. While these interactions are complex, they do demonstrate some discernible possibilities for intervention, some of which are already being systematically applied and some of which lend themselves more to individualized attention to a patient. The paradigm of stress-illness we have discussed will likely continue to serve well in the development of treatment programs and individualized patient care.

STRESS-RELATED ILLNESS

We have already discussed the current evidence for relationships between stressing life events and illness in general
and between stressing life events and illnesses commonly
classified as psychophysiological. Evidence for a relationship
between life stressors and other specific illnesses is more
tenuous, but we will now look at some illnesses about which
questions regarding the influence of stress have been asked.

IMMUNE-RELATED ILLNESSES

As you will recall, Selye's original concept of the biological
stress response involved an immunosuppressive effect. Mason
et al. (1979) showed how infectious disease could be
associated with hormonal responses generally related to stress.

Stressors of varying kinds affect the immune system in ways
that tend to make it less effective, thus possibly increasing
susceptibility to infection or hastening death from tumor im-
plantation (Miller, 1980). Such interactions are not surprising,
given the general impairment in bodily defenses that results
from an increase in the circulating steroids, as we mentioned in
Chapter 2. However, the responsiveness of the immune system
to psychological stimuli or to physiological mediators of their
exact effects on body functioning is not yet fully understood.

At present, there seems to be no doubt that stress is related to immune responsivity, but there is evidence that stress can relate to hypersensitivity as well as to hyposensitivity (Monjan and Collector, 1977). In an excellent review of the research on this relationship, Rogers, Dubey, and Reich (1979) described the methodological difficulties involved in immune research and the hazards they pose in trying to answer stress-related questions. For example, they pointed out that although excess amounts of steroids are known to be immunosuppressive, physiologically normal levels of corticosteroids are required for adequate immune functioning. The data on the influence of stress in areas of immune functioning such as killer-cell activity or interferon production are not always uniform. The suppression of functioning in T-lymphocytes, which are actually related to thymus functioning (an organ long known to be affected by stress) may have different manifestations depending on whether helper or suppressor T cells, which in turn regulate B lymphocytes, are affected. Rogers et al. (1979, p. 154) emphasized that the immune system is a complex network, subject to individual organismic differences such as cyclical variation: "It is important to avoid simplistic notions of stress and psychological experience as the "cause" of disease but rather as having a complex interaction with the personality and biology of the host and hence with the expression of disease." Amkraut and Solomon (1975) assessed the impact of stress on immune-related diseases such as bacterial disease, viral disease, cancer, autoimmune diseases, and allergic diseases. In general, they found that stress did have deleterious effects on these illnesses, but those effects were complex and interactive.

A very recent, excellent review of this area by Riley (1981) emphasizes that many of the difficulties in understanding these relationships are due to problems in experimental design. These difficulties have to do with whether an actual disease process is indeed susceptible to immune system influence, how the disease process interacts with the animal host, what initial levels of immune-related activity are under non-stress conditions, and so on. Riley (1981, p. 1109) concludes: "The forces of stress are limited, and in many circumstances are unable to exert any significant pathological effects. In other cases, however, the physiological and hormonal changes induced by emotional or anxiety stress are capable of shifting an immunological equipoise to produce lethal consequences." His conclusions are meant to apply to certain immune-related cancerous tumors as well as to immune-related infectious diseases. However, the experiments on which his observations are based were primarily animal in nature and it is unclear how completely the results will translate to human responses; nevertheless, the careful work he cites suggests there will be considerable transfer.

In sum, stress appears to have generally immunosuppressive effects with related illness consequences. However, the nature of these effects remains unclear.

CANCER

Stress-related factors that seem to have an effect on the development of cancer range from the loss of major emotional relationships (LeShan and Worthington, 1956; LeShan, 1959) and general psychosocial trauma (Paloucek and Graham, 1966; Greene and Swisher, 1969) to changes in hormonal activities, such as the production of 17-OHCS (Bulbrock and Hayward, 1967; Sholiton, Wohl, and Werk, 1963; Kissen and Rao, 1969). In a more recent study, Horne and Picard (1979) reported that retrospective identification of psychosocial risk factors such as job stability and recent loss of significant others could be used to correctly predict the diagnosis of benign (80 percent correct) and cancerous (61 percent correct) lung lesions in a population of 110 male patients with undiagnosed x-ray–identified lesions of the lung, while Scurry and Levin (1978) suggested that a lack of family closeness was related to the incidence of cancer. Rogentine et al. (1979) reported that patients who denied difficulties and tended to suppress their feelings toward life adjustments had a greater risk of melanoma relapse one year after testing.

In general, most studies support the idea that increased life stressors are associated with the occurrence of cancer. However, given the large number of people who would have to be screened in order to find a sample that would eventually get cancer, most of these studies are retrospective in nature. That is, they generally compare cancer patients with non-cancer patients or look for common characteristics among cancer patients. Therefore, by their nature, such studies confound the possible illness-related life stressors with independent life stressors that might antedate the illness, a methodological problem we discussed in Chapter 5. Thus, while generally supportive evidence for a stress-cancer relationship in terms of life events does exist, it is by no means conclusive.

The work of Riley (1981) cited earlier provides good evidence that certain immune-related tumors are susceptible to the effects of stress in an animal-experimentation model. Necessarily, stressors can be much better controlled and the constitutional characteristics of the animals and the specificity of type of tumor can be better identified in such situations. Sklar and Anisman (1981), in an extensive review of the literature, have extended the implications of animal research findings to humans in a theoretical sense. Their conclusion is not that stress can cause tumors, but that it can influence the "course of neoplastic disease" (p. 395) through its demonstrated influence on neurochemical, hormonal, and immunologic functioning.

Prospective studies of the influence of stress on subsequent tumor development in humans will need to be carried out before the clinical implications of any such relationship can be clarified. At present, the evidence suggest that such a relationship will probably prove to be of considerable importance when confirmed by future research.

RHEUMATOID ARTHRITIS

Rheumatoid arthritis is a chronic, systemic inflammatory disease of unknown cause. Its onset is usually insidious, but it can have an acute presentation when triggered by a stressing situation such as trauma, infection, or emotional upset. An associated immunopathology has also been found in rheumatoid arthritis patients, though its cause is still unclear.

Weiner (1977) reviewed studies of psychological characteristics of rheumatoid arthritis patients and suggested that stressing life events such as separation from a loved one, marital adjustment difficulties, birth, and death, as well as general emotional strain seem to be associated with the disease. There has also been some evidence that rheumatoid arthritis patients show increased muscular tension, especially near the affected joints.

The evidence for arthritis being a stress-related illness is intriguing, but again largely correlational; that is, the association has been demonstrated but causality has not been proven. Because of its association with a number of potentially stressing emotional events, and because of its association with immune-system disturbance, it is possible that stress plays a significant part in the development and manifestation of illness. However, the relationship must be described as speculative at this time.

GRAVE'S DISEASE (HYPERTHYROIDISM)

Grave's Disease, or hyperthyroidism, usually leads to forms of thyrotoxicosis associated with restlessness, nervousness, fatigue, and unexplained weight loss. It is one of the most common endocrine disorders. The illness basically involves a disruption of the regulatory processes of the thyroid and has long been thought to be associated with psychological factors (Weiner, 1977).

Weiner points out that Grave's Disease runs in families and may well involve constitutional predisposition. It has been associated with increased stress due to war, personal frustration and threat, worrying and grief, and surgical stress. However, because the illness is difficult to detect until acute manifestation occurs, it is almost impossible to tell whether stressing situations only aggravate the more blatant symptoms of the disease or contribute to the disease itself. Astwood (1967) reported that 50 percent of a group of patients with Grave's Disease had experienced personal life changes prior to onset of the disorder.

It is all the more plausible that there should be a relationship between stress and Grave's Disease, since the disease directly involves the endocrine system, which we already know to be involved in the basic stress response. (Thyroid secretion is controlled primarily by thyrotropin released by the pituitary.) However, even in this illness, the evidence for the relationship with stress is purely associational and not causal. We do not know whether stress-related hormonal responses cause or aggravate the illness itself or are merely corollary to it. For example, certain thyroid abnormalities can be detected in individuals who, though they may be at increased risk for thyroid disease, may never develop it (Weiner, 1977). It may be that such abnormalities reflect a predisposition that requires stress to activate its pathological consequences. With stress absent, either because there are no significant stressors or because coping has been efficient, there is no "trigger" for the disease. These theories are, of course, unproven.

PSYCHOLOGICAL DISTURBANCES

In Chapter 5, we discussed how life stressors have been

associated with increased psychological disturbances, ranging from simple neuroses to conditions requiring psychiatric hospitalization. Paykel (1978) confirmed that there is an increased risk of psychiatric illness following life stress, the risk being greater for depression and neurosis than for schizophrenia, and even more significant for suicide attempts. Schless, Teichman, Mendels, and DiGiacomo (1977) have suggested that life stress is a more significant risk factor for psychiatric illness than for medical illness, which in turn is associated with a higher incidence of life stress than is present in a "normal" population. Not all researchers have found such relationships, however. Hornstra and Klassen (1977) reported no increased relationship between life stress and depression, and Rabkin (1980) concluded that there was no increase in life stress among schizophrenics when compared with other patient groups.

Differences among studies of stress and psychological disturbance may be attributable to differences in research methodology, many of which have been reviewed by Paykel (1978). The use of different measures of life stress and psychiatric symptoms and different criteria for psychiatric diagnosis makes comparisons difficult. However, in clinical practice the occurrence of psychological crises has long been linked to the occurrence of various environmental events, even though the classification of such events may have been poorly developed. The work of Leavitt et al. discussed earlier suggested that, at least in back-pain patients, there was a relationship between the manifestation of illness, psychological disturbance, and life stress, when these relationships were measured in a straightforward, quantitative manner.

Horowitz (1976) termed specific psychological responses to stressors the "stress response syndrome." Basically, this syndrome is the time-related development of a response following the onset of a stressor. After someone experiences a stressing event, there is usually a reflex emotional expression that is followed by a tendency to deny the occurrence of the event. Later, thoughts about the stressor intrude, characterized by nonvolitional ideas, feelings about the stressor, dreams about the event, and mixed interpretations about the meaning of the event and its influence on other aspects of life. Eventually, the individual adapts to the stressor and accepts its occurrence, gradually coming to a personal resolution of the stress associated with the event.

Much of Horowitz's conceptualization is similar to classical mourning theory, which deals with the course of events following the death of a close relative or friend. He is probably correct in applying this concept to the occurrence of major stressors like medical illness and the resulting loss of occupational function and status. This approach is useful in that it helps us identify significant aspects of stressor occurrence and coping responses. However, the process is probably not peculiar to stress situations alone. To date, no specific emotional or behavioral stress response has been identified nor should we expect to find one, since individual coping styles are so varied.

The evidence for a relationship between stress and psychiatric illness has many methodological and conceptual weaknesses, which is not surprising given the highly individual nature of psychological functioning (Bieliauskas, 1981). At an individual level, however, our stress-illness paradigm will probably provide useful information about responses to stressors and the role these responses play in the development of psychological disturbances.

CONCLUSIONS

As noted at the beginning of this chapter, the evidence relating stress to specific illnesses is weak, and in many ways, unconvincing. This is mainly due to variations in the research methodologies that have been used in investigating relation-ships. However, I believe the enormous quantity of anecdotal and correlational evidence is difficult to ignore and I have found that in clinical practice attention to stress-related factors frequently proves to be beneficial in patient treatment. Future research will hinge on the continued development of research designs and techniques that will specify the magnitude, nature, and direction of the stress-illness relationship.

STRESS, HEALTH, AND ILLNESS: A SUMMARY

Is stress related to illness? The answer appears to be "yes," but the strength of the relationship has not been clearly demonstrated. Nor do our current findings provide a sound basis for consistent, accurate predictions of the course of illness or for effective intervention in the illness process. The reason a strong relationship has not been demonstrated at this time is likely related to the complexity that has become evident in examining variables of stressors, mediating factors, stress, and coping. It is clear that each of the components of the stress-illness paradigm may have individual variations and may depend on past experience with stressors, the social and psychological context of a stressor and the individual at a given time, the individual variability of hormonal patterns, and individual coping abilities. The full stress-illness paradigm we developed was:

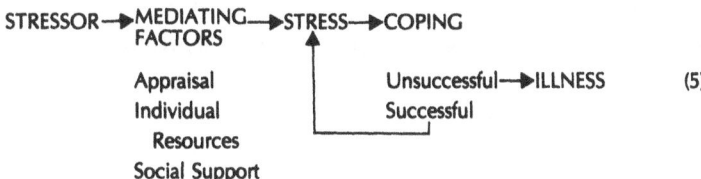

$$(5)$$

As I have defined the term, "stress" refers to the biological and psychological response to a stressor. Not all authors would

agree with this definition; some prefer to label significant life events as "stress," rather than as "stressors." I think this leads to confusion between the stimulus and response aspects of given situations; events can easily be misidentified and the resulting conceptualization of responses to those events will be equally muddled. If the components of a stress-illness paradigm are kept distinct, we can more effectively identify what it is we are referring to when we say that an event is stressing or that a category of behavior is a method of coping with stress.

At the start of this volume, I noted that Selye's General Adaptation Syndrome described the sequence of a stress response. The GAS still appears to have validity, not because there have been any clear demonstrations that it describes specific biological or psychological parameters, but because it makes sense in terms of what we know about how people react when confronted with a stressor stimulus. The immediate reaction is a mobilization of resources, followed by an extended period during which adaptation is made to living with a stressor when immediate defenses do not work, and then eventual breakdown (illness) when the strength to continue adaptation wanes. The GAS provides an accurate general description although, as I have pointed out many times, the true stress response embraces a multitude of intervening psychological and biological factors.

Time seems to be a particularly important factor in whether or not a stressor ultimately produces a stress response. If a person's initial cognitive appraisal of a stressor changes so that the event is no longer perceived as a stressor, then obviously that stimulus no longer falls within our stress-illness paradigm. Similarly, the presence of social mediators in the stress-illness paradigm will mitigate the threatening nature of a stressor and also reduce or short-circuit a stress response; an example of this would be the presence of a supportive family atmosphere to which one can return from a stressing daytime occupation, where the need for continued adaptation can be "forgotten" during the evening. Finally, effective coping skills, whether already present or learned as needed, can also change the nature of a stressor from threatening to challenging or even exciting. The importance of all these factors has been tested in the studies we cited. It is only after appraisal, support, and coping have failed to deal with a stressor effectively that the stress response takes place over time and eventually leads to illness.

The complexity of the stress response makes it seem almost impossible to generate a theory that will cover all the important aspects of stress-illness relationships. Burchfield (1979, p. 669) has made an elegant attempt to integrate this diversity into a stress-response theory. She states that:

> organisms are predisposed to adapt to chronic intermittent stress. Adaptation is achieved by anticipation of the stressor and decreased responsivity. These are expressed physiologically as a conditioned endocrine response to environmental stimuli predictive of the stressor, and a decreasing arousal response after stressor onset. Maladaptation is manifested as an increased or maintained arousal response occasionally continuing to occur despite the absence of a stressor. Failure to adapt may be due to any number of variables . . . but is hypothesized to be due most often to learned cognitive states . . . rather than stressor exposure *per se,* the maladaptive response to stress is responsible for the increased illness susceptibility frequently found to follow stress.

Burchfield's views are generally consistent with the evidence we have presented on how stressors are perceived, reacted to, and coped with. The belief that most individuals are geared to successfully adapt to stressors is in keeping with the fact that if stressors are taken literally as stimuli that tax the resources of an individual, then we are all coping with stressors in some way most of the time and doing a fairly good job of it. Antonovsky's

(1979) proposition that we should focus on promoting health rather than on explaining illness relied on the notion that the stress-illness relationship reflected some failure in an otherwise adequate repertoire of appraisal, support, coping skills, and resources. It is clear that from this perspective research that is limited to studying illnesses following the occurrence of stressors necessarily ignores the broader range of interactive factors that we have described, and thus fails to demonstrate strong stress-illness relationships.

From a medical treatment standpoint, the task of delineating important aspects of how stress may relate to illness in the individual case involves the following questions:

1. Is a stressor present, either externally (such as a threatening event) or internally (such as a fear of failure at work)? If so, should treatment involve attempts to alter the presence of the stressor temporarily or permanently, by taking a vacation or changing jobs, for example?
2. Does the patient have an accurate appraisal of the stressor—is his perception of a stimulus or event accurate? For example, is a generally good student interpreting his inability to complete a given academic course as an overall personal failure? If so, attempts can be made to modify that appraisal through counseling or therapy.
3. Does the patient have an effective social support system? Without such support, threat may have deleterious effects. If support can be rallied by consultation with, for example, family members, the effects of the stressor may be eased. For instance, suppose a patient has become irritable, unpersonable, and easily fatigued after suffering a closed-head injury. The patient's family may think he is being lazy, aloof,

and irascible, and treat him in a hostile fashion. Explaining that the patient is experiencing a post-traumatic syndrome may change the family's perception, increasing understanding and support for the patient and speeding recovery.

4. Is the individual actually experiencing a stress response? This question cannot always be answered straightforwardly. Hormonal assays might give us clues, but hormonal levels alone are not enough given current evidence, nor are such tests practical in terms of cost/benefit ratios. Personal reports of anxiety, fear, and discomfort may actually provide better clues. A patient voicing such complaints should be considered at risk for developing illness and should be monitored as long as the stress continues especially if a tendency toward specific illness patterns exists (such as a history of asthma attacks).

5. Does the patient have a history of maladjustment, either physical or psychological? Such persons appear to be at higher risk than others of developing illness in response to stressors.

6. Does the individual live in a high-stress situation? Is there an environment of heightened social, family, or occupational stressors? Such persons also appear to be at higher risk for developing illness in response to a stressor.

7. If the patient is suffering from a specifically caused illness, such as a viral infection, is he or she also experiencing a stress response to other aspects of the environment? Crossed-sensitization should be considered if this is the case, and attempts should be made to deal with the additional contributor to the stress response.

8. Does the individual possess effective coping

resources? Can he or she deal with what is perceived as being threatening? If not, we can try to increase coping abilities through education or training and help the individual to realize the full extent of available coping resources. If the individual feels unable to control or predict events, we should also try to maximize the individual's sense of control and help him predict the course of whatever illness or other stressor he is facing.

We have outlined some methods of modifying the stress-illness interaction in this volume, but only in a cursory fashion. A much fuller treatment of intervention approaches in health care is given by Gordon (1981) in another volume in this series.

Antonovsky (1979), whose theory of health maintenance is based on a sense of "coherence" with one's environment, offered several guidelines for avoiding common pitfalls in medical care. First, he suggested that the patient's sense of coherence is impaired if all decision making is left in the hands of medical personnel. A physician or nurse cannot always be around to attend to a patient's needs and the patient should not be made to feel helpless without a caretaker at his side. Otherwise, those instances when immediate care is not available will be particularly stressing. Second, Antonovsky suggested that we often ignore the cultural context from which our patients come, which in the United States, tends to equate participation in determining goals to be achieved with decisional input. If the medical practitioner is viewed as omnipotent, which is seldom the case, this will violate the need of many patients to have some say in what is done to them and lead to a sense of lack of coherence. Third, no medical practitioner can summarily suspend all other commitments beyond the immediate needs of a single patient; there are other patient responsibilities and needs for financial solvency. The more a patient perceives the practitioner's behavior as not being in his or her total interest, the greater the lack of coherence for the patient. This does not mean restructuring reality to meet the expectations of commitment in patients; rather we must try to explain what we do and why we do it so that the patient's fears of being uncared for, or even of being exploited, can be put to rest.

In closing, I can reaffirm the importance of Antonovsky's cautions and suggestions. The more we become aware of the relationships between stress, illness, and health, the better we will be at treating illness and, ultimately, in working to promote health.

BIBLIOGRAPHY

Aldrich, C.K., and Mendkoff, E. "Relocation of the aged and disabled: A mortality study." *Journal of the American Geriatric Society,* 1963, 11:185–194.

Alexander, A.B. "Chronic asthma." In R.B. Williams and W.B. Gentry (eds.), *Behavioral approaches to medical treatment.* Cambridge, Massachusetts: Ballinger Publishing Company, 1977.

Alexander, F.G., and Selesnick, S.T. *The history of psychiatry.* New York: Harper and Row, 1966.

Amkraut, A., and Solomon, G.F. "From the symbolic stimulus to the pathophysiological response: Immune mechanisms." *International Journal of Psychiatry in Medicine,* 1975, 5:541–563.

Antonovsky, A. *Health, stress, and coping.* Washington: Jossey-Bass, 1979.

Aponte, J.J., and Miller, F.T. "Stress-related social events and psychological impairment." *Journal of Clinical Psychology,* 1972, 28:455–458.

Astwood, E.B. "Use of antithyroid drugs." In W.J. Irvine (ed.), *Thyrotoxicosis.* Edinburgh: Livingstone, 1967.

Batlis, N., Webb, J.T., Dekker, D., and Muelheisen, R. "The relationship of stressful life events and hospitalization in a student sample." Paper presented at the meeting of the Ohio Psychological Association, 1972, Columbus, Ohio.

Baxter, J.D., and Rousseau, G.G. *Glucocorticoid hormone action.* New York: Springer, 1979.

Belar, C.D. "A comment on Silver and Blanchard's (1978) review of the treatment of tension headaches in EMG feedback and relaxation training." *Journal of Behavioral Medicine*, 1978, 2:215–220.

Benson, H., Marzetta, B.R., and Rosner, B.A. "Decreased blood pressure associated with the regular elicitation of relaxation response: A study of hypertensive subjects." In R.S. Eliot (ed.), *Stress and the heart*. New York: Futura, 1974.

Bieliauskas, L.A. "Life events, 17-OHCS measures, and psychological defensiveness in relation to aid-seeking." *Journal of Human Stress*, 1980, 6:28–36.

_____. *The influence of individual differences in health and illness*. Boulder, Colorado: Westview Press, 1981.

Bieliauskas, L.A., and Strugar, D.A. "Sample size characteristics and scores on the Social Readjustment Rating Scale." *Journal of Psychosomatic Research*, 1976, 20:201–205.

Bieliauskas, L.A., and Webb, J.T. "The social readjustment rating scale: validity in a college population." *Journal of Psychosomatic Research*, 1974, 18:115–123.

Bing, E. *Six practical lessons for an easier childbirth*. New York: Bantam Books, 1969.

Bliss, E.L., Migeon, C.J., Branch, C.H., and Samuels, L.T. "Reaction of the adrenal cortex to emotional stress." *Psychosomatic Medicine*, 1956, 18:56–76.

Blix, A.S., Stromme, S.B., and Ursin, H. "Additional heart rate – an indicator of psychological activation." *Aerospace Medicine*, 1974, 45:1219–1222.

Blumenthal, J.A., Williams, R.S., Williams, R.B., and Wallace, A.G. "Effects of exercise on Type A (coronary prone) behavior pattern." *Psychosomatic Medicine*, 1980, 42:289–296.

Brady, J. "Ulcers in executive monkeys." *Scientific American*, 1958, 199:362–404.

Budzynski, T.H. "Clinical implications of electromyographic training." In G.E. Schwartz and J. Beatty (eds.), *Biofeedback, theory and research*. New York: Academic Press, 1977.

Bulbrock, R.D., and Hayward, J.L. "Abnormal urinary steroid excretion and subsequent breast cancer." *Lancet*, March 11, 1967: 591–522.

Burchfield, S.R. "The stress response: A new perspective." *Psychosomatic Medicine*, 1979, 41:661–672.

Caplan, J. *Support systems and community mental health.* New York: Behavioral Publications, 1974.

Caplan, R.D. "A less heretical view of life change and hospitalization." *Journal of Psychosomatic Research*, 1975, 19:247–250.

Carlson, L.A. "Pharmacological control of free fatty acid mobilization and plasma triglyceride transport." In R.J. Jones (ed.), *Atherosclerosis, Proceedings of the Second International Symposium.* Berlin: Springer, 1970.

Carter, H., and Glick, P.C. *Marriage and divorce: A social and economic study.* Cambridge, Massachusetts: Harvard University Press, 1970.

Casey, R.L., Masuda, M., and Holmes, T.H. "Quantitative study of recall of life events." *Journal of Psychosomatic Research*, 1967, 11:239–247.

Cassel, J. "Social science in epidemiology: Psychosocial processes and "stress", theoretical correlation." In E. Streuning and M. Guttentag (eds.), *Handbook of evaluation research.* Beverly Hills, California: Sage, 1975.

Cassens, G., Roffman, M., Kuruc, A., Orsulak, P.J., and Schildkraut, J.J. "Alterations in brain norepinephrine metabolism induced by environmental stimuli previously paired with inescapable shock." *Science*, 1980, 209:1138–1140.

Chan, K.B. "Individual differences in reactions to stress and their personality and situational determinants: Some implications for community mental health." *Social Science and Medicine*, 1977, 11:89–103.

Chiriboga, D.A., and Dean, H. "Dimensions of stress: Perspectives from a longitudinal study." *Journal of Psychosomatic Research*, 1978, 22:47–55.

Cline, D.W., and Chosey, J.J. "A prospective study of life changes and subsequent health changes." *Archives of General Psychiatry*, 1972, 27:51–53.

Cobb, S. Physiological changes in men whose jobs were eliminated." *Journal of Psychosomatic Research*, 1974, 18:245–258.

Cohen, J.J., McArthur, D.L., and Rickles, W.H. "Comparison of four biofeedback treatments for migraine headache: Physiological and headache variables." *Psychosomatic Medicine,* 1980, 42:463–480.

Cooper, M.J., and Aygen, M.M. "A relaxation technique in the management of hypercholesterolemia." *Journal of Human Stress,* 1979, 5:23–36.

Counte, M.A., and Christman, L.P. *Interpersonal behavior and health care.* Boulder, Colorado: Westview Press, 1981.

Crandall, J.E., and Lehman, R.E. "Relationship of stressful life events to social interest." *Journal of Consulting and Clinical Psychology,* 1977, 145:1208.

Croog, S.H., and Fitzgerald, E.F. "Subjective stress and serious illness of a spouse: Wives of heart patients." *Journal of Health and Social Behavior,* 1978, 19:166–178.

Dahlstrom, W.G., Welsh, G.S., and Dahlstrom, L.E. *An MMPI handbook, volume 1: Clinical interpretation.* Minneapolis: University of Minnesota Press, 1972.

Dalessio, D.J. (ed.). *Wolff's headache and other head pain.* New York: Oxford Press, 1972.

Dean, A., and Lin, N. "The stress-buffering role of social support: Problems and prospectives for systematic investigation." *Journal of Nervous and Mental Disease,* 1977, 165:403–407.

Dekker, D.J., and Webb, J.T. "Relationships of the Social Readjustment Rating Scale to psychiatric patient status, anxiety, and social desirability." *Journal of Psychosomatic Research,* 1974, 18:125–130.

Dembroski, J.M., MacDougall, J.M., and Lushene, R. "Interpersonal interaction and cardiovascular response in Type A subjects and coronary patients." *Journal of Human Stress,* 1979, 4:28–36.

Dimsdale, J.E., and Moss, J.M. "Short-term catecholamine response to psychological stress." *Psychosomatic Medicine,* 1980, 42:493–497.

Dohrenwend, B.P. "Problems in defining and sampling the relevant population of stressful life events." In B.S. Dohrenwend and B.P. Dohrenwend (eds.), *Stressful life events: Their nature and effects.* New York: Wiley, 1974.

Dohrenwend, B.S., and Dohrenwend, B.P. "Some issues in research on stressful life events." *Journal of Nervous and Mental Disease,* 1978, 166:7–15.

Dohrenwend, B.S., Krasnoff, L., Askenasy, A.R., and Dohrenwend, B.P. "Exemplification of a method for scaling life events: The PERI life events scale." *Journal of Health and Social Behavior,* 1978, 19:205–229.

Dougherty, T.F. "Some observations on mechanisms of corticosteroid action on inflammatory and immunologic processes." *Annals of the New York Academy of Sciences,* 1953, 56:748–756.

Faris, R., and Dunham, H. *Mental disorders in urban areas.* Chicago: University of Chicago Press, 1939.

Fordtran, J.S. "Acid secretion in peptic ulcer." In M.H. Sleisenger and J.S. Fordtran (eds.), *Gastrointestinal disease.* Philadelphia: Saunders, 1973.

Fordyce, W.E. *Behavioral methods for chronic pain and illness.* St. Louis: Mosby, 1976.

Frankenhauser, M. "Psychoneuroendocrine approaches to the study of stressful person-environment transactions." In H. Selye (ed.), *Selye's guide to stress research, volume I.* New York: Van Nostrand, 1980.

Friedman, M., and Rosenman, R.H. *Type A behavior and your heart.* New York: Knopf, 1974.

_____. "Modification of the Type A coronary-prone behavior pattern." Paper presented at the meeting of the American Psychological Association, 1977, San Francisco.

Garrity, T.F., Marx, M.B., and Somes, G.W. "The influence of illness severity and time since life change on the size of the life change–health change relationship." *Journal of Psychosomatic Research,* 1977, 21:377–382.

Gentry, W.D., and Bernal, G.A.A. "Chronic pain." In R.B. Williams and W.D. Gentry (eds.), *Behavioral approaches to medical treatment.* Cambridge, Massachusetts: 1977.

Gersten, J.C., Langner, T.S., Eisenberg, J.G., and Orzek, L. "Child behavior and life events: Undesirable change or change per se." In B.S. Dohrenwend and B.P. Dohrenwend (eds.), *Stressful life events: Their nature and effects.* New York: Wiley, 1974.

Glass, D.C. "Stress, behavior patterns, and coronary disease." *American Scientist,* 1977, 65:177–187.

Glass, D.C., Singer, J.E., and Friedman, L.N. "Psychic cost of adaptation to environmental stressors." *Journal of Personality and Social Psychology,* 1969, 12:200–210.

Gordon, L.B. *Behavioral intervention in health care.* Boulder, Colorado: Westview Press, 1981.

Greene, W.A., and Swisher, S.N. "Psychological and somatic variables associated with the development and course of monozygotic twins discordant for leukemia." *Annals of the New York Academy of Sciences,* 1969, 164:394–407.

Handlon, J.H., Wadeson, R.W., Fishman, J.R., Sachar, E.J., Hamburg, D.A., and Mason, J.W. "Psychological factors lowering 17-hydroxycorticosteroid concentration." *Psychosomatic Medicine,* 1962, 24:535–542.

Harmon, D.K., Masuda, M., and Holmes, T.H. "The Social Readjustment Rating Scale: A cross-cultural study of Western Europeans and Americans." *Journal of Psychosomatic Research,* 1970, 14:391–400.

Haynes, S.N., Griffin, P., Mooney, D., and Parise, M. "Electromyographic feedback and relaxation instructions in the treatment of muscle contraction headache." *Behavioral Therapy,* 1975, 6: 672–678.

Henry, J.P. "Understanding the early pathophysiology of essential hypertension." *Geriatrics,* 1976, 33:59–72.

Hetzel, B.S., Schottstaedt, W.W., Grace, W.J., and Wolff, H.G. "Changes in urinary 17-hydroxycorticosteroid excretion during stressful life situations in man." *Journal of Clinical Endocrinology,* 1955, 15:1057–1068.

Hill, S.R., Goetz, F.C., Fox, H.M., Murawski, B.J., Krakauer, L.J., Reifenstein, R.W., Gray, S.J., Reddy, W.J., Hedberg, S.E., St. Marc, J.R., and Thorn, G.W. "Studies on adrenocortical and psychological responses to stress in man." *Archives of Internal Medicine,* 1956, 97:269–298.

Hinkle, L.E. "The effect of exposure to cultural change, social change, and changes in interpersonal relationships in health." In B.S.

Dohrenwend and B.P. Dohrenwend (eds.), *Stressful life events: Their nature and effects.* New York: Wiley, 1974.

Hock, R.A., Rodgers, C.H., Reddi, C., and Kennard, D.W. "Medico-psychological intervention in male asthmatic children: An evaluation of physiological change." *Psychosomatic Medicine,* 1978, 40:210–215.

Hodges, J.R., Jones, M.T., and Stockham, M.A. "Effect of emotion on blood corticotrophins and cortisol concentrations in man." *Nature,* 1962, 193:1187.

Hofer, M.A., Wolff, C.T., Friedman, S.B., and Mason, J.W. "A psychoendocrine study of bereavement, Part I. 17-hydroxy-corticosteroid excretion rates of parents following death of their children from leukemia." *Psychosomatic Medicine,* 1972, 34:481–491.

Holmes, T.S., and Holmes, T.H. "Short term intrusions in the life style routine." *Journal of Psychosomatic Research,* 1970, 14:121–132.

Holmes, T.H., and Masuda, M. "Life change and illness suscep-tibility." In B.S. Dohrenwend and B.P. Dohrenwend (eds.), *Stressful life events: Their nature and effects.* New York: Wiley, 1974.

Holmes, T.H., and Rahe, R.H. "The Social Readjustment Rating Scale." *Journal of Psychosomatic Research,* 1967, 11:213–218.

Hornstra, R.K., and Klassen, D. "The course of depression." *Comprehensive Psychiatry,* 1977, 18:119–125.

Horowitz, M.J. *Stress response syndromes.* New York: Aronson, 1976.

Horowitz, M., Wilner, B.A., and Alvarez, W. "Impact of events scale: A measure of subjective stress." *Psychosomatic Medicine,* 1979, 41:209–218.

Horne, R.L., and Picard, R.S. "Psychosocial risk factors for lung cancer." *Psychosomatic Medicine,* 1979, 41:503–514.

Hudgens, R.W. "Personal catastrophe and depression: A considera-tion of the subject with respect to medically ill adolescents, and a requiem for retrospective life-event studies." In B.S. Dohren-wend and B.P. Dohrenwend (eds.), *Stressful life events: Their nature and effects.* New York: Wiley, 1974.

Ingle, D.J. "Permissive action of hormones." *Journal of Clinical Endo-*

crinology, 1954, 14:1272–1274.

Jenkins, C.D. "Psychosocial modifiers of response to stress." *Journal of Human Stress,* 1979, 5:3–15.

Jenkins, C.D., Zyzanski, S.J., and Rosenman, R.H. *Manual for the Jenkins Activity Survey.* New York: Psychological Corporation, 1979.

Jenkins, C.D., Zyzanski, S.J., Ryan, T.J., Flessas, A., and Tannenbaum, S.I. "Social insecurity and coronary-prone Type A responses as identifiers of severe atherosclerosis." *Journal of Consulting and Clinical Psychology,* 1977, 45:1060–1067.

Kasl, S.V., Evans, A.S., and Niederman, J.C. "Psychosocial risk factors and infectious mononucleosis." *Psychosomatic Medicine,* 1979, 41:455–465.

Katz, J., Weiner, H., Gallagner, T., and Hellman, L. "Stress, distress, and ego defenses." *Archives of General Psychiatry,* 1970, 23:131–142.

Kinsman, R.A., Dirks, J.F., Jones, N.F., and Dahlem, N.W. "Anxiety reduction in asthma: From catches to general application." *Psychosomatic Medicine,* 1980, 42:397–406.

Kiritz, S., and Moos, R.H. "Physiological effects of social environments." *Psychosomatic Medicine,* 1974, 36:96–114.

Kissen, D.M., and Rao, L.G.S. "Steroid excretion patterns and personality in lung cancer." *Annals of the New York Academy of Sciences,* 1969, 164:476–482.

Klein, R.F., Kliner, V.A., Zipes, D.P., Troyer, W.G., and Wallace, A.G. "Transfer from a coronary care unit." *Archives of Internal Medicine,* 1968, 122:104–108.

Kolb, L.C. *Modern clinical psychiatry.* Philadelphia: Saunders, 1973.

Komaroff, A.L., Masuda, M., and Holmes, T.H. "The Social Readjustment Rating Scale: A comparative study of negro, Mexican, and white Americans." *Journal of Psychosomatic Research,* 1968, 12:121–128.

Lacey, J.I. "Somatic response patterning and stress: Some revisions of activation theory." In M.H. Appley and R. Trumbull (eds.), *Psychological stress.* New York: Appleton-Century-Crofts, 1967.

Lake, A., Rainey, J., and Papsdorf, J.D. "Biofeedback and rational-emotive therapy in the management of major headache." *Journal* of *Applied Behavior Analysis,* 1979, 12:127–140.

Lazarus, R.S. "Cognitive and coping processes in emotion." In A. Monat and R.S. Lazarus (eds.), *Stress and coping: An anthology.* New York: Columbia University Press, 1977.

Lazarus, R.S., Cohen, J.B., Folkman, S., Kanner, A., and Schaefer, C. "Psychological stress and adaptation: Some unresolved issues." In H. Selye (ed.), *Selye's guide to stress research, volume I.* New York: Van Nostrand, 1980.

Leavitt, F., Garron, D.C., and Bieliauskas, L.A. "Stressing life events and the experience of low back pain." *Journal of Psychosomatic Research,* 1979, 23:149–154.

———. "Psychological disturbance and life event differences among patients with low back pain." *Journal of Consulting and Clinical Psychology,* 1980, 48:115–116.

Leavitt, F., Garron, D.C., Whisler, W.W., and Sheinkop, M.B. "Affective and sensory dimensions of low back pain." *Pain,* 1978, 4:273–281.

Lehrer, S. "Life change and gastric cancer." *Psychosomatic medicine,* 1980, 42:499–502.

LeShan, L. "Psychological states as factors in the development of malignant disease: A critical review." *Journal of the National Cancer Institute,* 1959, 22:1–18.

LeShan, L., and Worthington, R.D. "Some recurrent life history patterns observed in patients with malignant disease." *Journal of Nervous and Mental Disease,* 1956, 124:460–465.

Lief, A. (ed.) *The commonsense psychiatry of Dr. Adolph Meyer.* New York: McGraw-Hill, 1948.

Lin, N., Simeone, R., Ensel, W., and Kuo, W. "Social support, stressful life events, and illness: A model and an empirical test." *Journal of Health and Social Behavior,* 1979, 20:108–119.

Maddison, D., and Walker, W.L. "Factors affecting the outcome of conjugal bereavement." *British Journal of Psychiatry,* 1967, 113:1057–1067.

Manogue, K.R., Leshner, A.I., and Candland, D.K. "Dominance status and adrenocortical activity to stress in squirrel monkeys (Saimiri Sciureus)." *Primates,* 1975, 16:457–463.

Marcussen, R.M., and Wolff, H.G. "A formulation of the dynamics of the migraine attack." *Psychosomatic Medicine,* 1949, 11:251–256.

Mason, J.W. "Psychological influences on the pituitary-adrenal cortical system." *Recent Progress in Hormone Research,* 1959a, 15:345–378.

_____. "Visceral function of the nervous system." *Annual Review of Physiology,* 1959b, 21:353–380.

_____. "A review of psychoendocrine research on the pituitary adrenal system." *Psychosomatic Medicine,* 1968, 30:576–607.

_____. "A re-evaluation of the concept of non-specificity in stress theory." *Journal of Psychiatric Research,* 1971, 8:323–333.

Mason, J.W., and Brady, J.V. "Plasma 17-hydroxicorticosteroid changes related to reserpine effects on emotional behaviors." *Science,* 1956, 124:983–984.

Mason, J.W., Buescher, E.L., Belfer, M.L, Artenstein, M.S., and Mougey, E.H. "A prospective study of corticosteroid and catecholamine levels in relation to viral respiratory illness." *Journal of Human Stress,* 1979, 5:18–28.

Mason, J.W., Maher, J.T., Hartley, L.H., Mougey, E., Perlow, M.H., and Jones, L.G. "Selectivity of corticosteroid and catecholamine response to various natural stimuli." In G. Serban (ed.), *Psychopathology of human adaptation.* New York: Plenum, 1976.

Masuda, M., and Holmes, T.H. "The Social Readjustment Rating Scale: A cross-cultural study of Japanese and Americans." *Journal of Psychosomatic Research,* 1967, 11:227–237.

Mechanic, D. "Stress, illness, and illness behavior." *Journal of Human Stress,* 1976, 2:2–6.

Mechanic, D. "Effects of psychological distress on perceptions of physical health and use of medical and psychiatric facilities." *Journal of Human Stress,* 1978, 4:26–33.

_____. "Effects of psychological distress on perception of physical health and use of medical and psychiatric facilities." *Journal of Human Stress,* 1980, 4:26–32.

Melzack, R., and Torgerson, W.S. "On the language of pain." *Anesthesiology,* 1971, 34:50–59.

Miller, N.E. "Effects of learning on physical symptoms produced by psychological stress." In H. Selye (ed.), *Selye's guide to stress research, volume I.* New York: Van Nostrand, 1980.

Monjan, A.A., and Collector, M.I. "Stress-induced modulation of the immune response." *Science,* 1977, 196:307–308.

Natelson, B.H., and Cagin, N.A. "Stress-induced ventricular arrhythmias." *Psychosomatic Medicine,* 1979, 41:259–262.

Nuckolls, K.B., Cassel, J., and Kaplan, B.H. "Psychosocial assets, life crisis, and the prognosis of pregnancy." *American Journal of Epidemiology,* 1972, 95:431–441.

Oken, D., Grinker, R.R., Heath, H.A., Herz, M., Korchin, S.H., Sabshin, M., and Schwartz, N.B. "Relation of physiological response to affective expression." *Archives of General Psychiatry,* 1962, 6:336–351.

Oliver, M.F. "Free fatty acid and the ischaemic myocardium." *Advances in cardiology,* 1974, 12:84–93.

Orth-Gomer, K., Ahlborn, A., and Theorell, T. "Impact of pattern A behavior on ischemic heart disease when controlling for conventional risk indicators." *Journal of Human Stress,* 1980, 6:6–13.

Palkovits, M., Kobayaski, P.M., Kizer, J., Jacobowitz, D.M., and Kopin, I.J. "Effects of stress on catecholamines and tyrosine hydroxylase activity of individual hypothalamic nuclei." *Neuroendocrinology,* 1975, 18:144–153.

Paloucek, F.P., and Graham, J.B. "The influence of psycho-social factors on the prognosis in cancer of the cervix." *Annals of the New York Academy of Sciences,* 1966, 125:814–816.

Paykel, E.S. "Contribution of life events to causation of psychiatric illness." *Psychological Medicine,* 1978, 8:245–253.

Paykel, E.S., Meyers, J.K., Dienelt, M.N., Klerman, C.L., Lindenthal, J.J., and Pepper, M.P. "Life events and depression." *Archives of General Psychiatry,* 1969, 21:753–760.

Poe, R.O., Rose, R.M., and Mason, J.W. "Multiple determinants of 17-hydroxycorticosteroid excretion in recruits during basic training." *Psychosomatic Medicine,* 1970, 32:369–378.

Pomerleau, O.F. "Behavioral medicine, the contribution of the experimental analysis of behavior to medical care." *American*

Psychologist, 1979, 34:654–663.

Rabkin, J.G. "Stressful life events and schizophrenia: A review of the research literature." *Psychological Bulletin,* 1980, 87:408–425.

Rabkin, J.G., and Streuning, E.L. "Life events, stress, and illness." *Science,* 1976, 194:1013–1020.

Rahe, R.H. "Multi-cultural correlations of life change scaling: America, Japan, Denmark, and Sweden." *Journal of Psychosomatic Research,* 1969, 13:191–195.

Rahe, R.H., and Arthur, R.J. "Life change and illness studies." *Journal of Human Stress,* 1978, 4:3–15.

Rahe, R.H., Mahan, J.J., and Arthur, R.J. "Prediction of near-future health changes from subjects' preceding life changes." *Journal of Psychosomatic Research,* 1970, 14:401–406.

Rahe, R.H., and Paasikivi, J. "Psychosocial factors and myocardial infarction, II: An outpatient study in Sweden." *Journal of Psychosomatic Research,* 1971, 15:33–39.

Redfield, J., and Stone, A. "Individual viewpoints of stressful life events." *Journal of Consulting and Clinical Psychology,* 1979, 47:147–154.

Reeder, L.G., Scharama, P.G.M., and Dirken, J.M. "Stress and cardiovascular health: An international cooperative study – I." *Social Sciences and Medicine,* 1973, 7:573–584.

Riley, V. "Psychoneuroendocrine influences on immunocompetence and neoplasia." *Science,* 1981, 212:1100–1109.

Rogentine, G.N., van Kammen, D.P., Fox, B.H., Docherty, J.P., Rosenblatt, J.E., Boyd, S.C., and Bunney, W.E. "Psychological factors in the prognosis of malignant melanoma: A prospective study." *Psychosomatic Medicine,* 1979, 41:647–655.

Rogers, M.P., Dubey, D., and Reich, P. "The influence of the psyche and the brain on immunity and disease susceptibility: A critical review." *Psychosomatic Medicine,* 1979, 41:147–164.

Rosenman, R.H., Brand, R.J., Jenkins, C.D., Friedman, M., Straus, R., and Wurm, M. "Coronary heart disease in the Western Collaborative Group Study: Final follow-up experience of 8½ years." *Journal of the American Medical Association,* 1975, 233:872–877.

Rosenman, R.H., and Friedman, M. "Neurogenic factors in pathogenesis of coronary heart disease." *Medical Clinics of North America,* 1974, 58:269–279.

Roskies, E., Kearney, H., Spevack, M., Surkis, A., Cohen, C., and Gilman, S. "Generalization and durability of treatment efforts in an intervention program for coronary-prone (Type A) managers." *Journal of Behavioral Medicine,* 1979, 2:195–207.

Roskies, E., Spevack, M., Surkis, A., Cohan, C., and Gilman, S. "Changing the coronary-prone (Type A) behavior pattern in a nonclinical population." *Journal of Behavioral Medicine,* 1978, 1:201–216.

Rubin, R.T., Gunderson, E.K.E., and Arthur, R.J. "Life stress and illness patterns in the U.S. Navy–V. Prior life change and illness onset in a battleship's crew." *Journal of Psychosomatic Research,* 1971, 15:89–94.

Ruch, L.O. "A multidimensional analysis of the concept of life change." *Journal of Health and Social Behavior,* 1977, 18:71–83.

Ruch, L.O., and Holmes, T.H. "Scaling of life change: Comparison of direct and indirect methods." *Journal of Psychosomatic Research,* 1971, 15:221–227.

Sarason, I.G., Johnson, J.H., and Siegel, J.M. "Assessing the impact of life changes: Development of the life experiences survey." *Journal of Consulting and Clinical Psychology,* 1978, 46:932–946.

Schless, A.P., Teichman, A., Mendels, J., and DiGiacomo, J.N. *British Journal of Psychiatry,* 1977, 130:19–22.

Schmale, A.H. "Giving up as a final common pathway to changes in health." *Advances in Psychosomatic Medicine,* 1972, 8:20–40.

Schwartz, G.E. "Biofeedback and patterning of autonomic and central processes: CNS-cardiovascular interactions." In G.E. Schwartz and J. Beatty (eds.), *Biofeedback, theory and research.* New York: Academic Press, 1977.

Scurry, M.T., and Levin, E.M. "Psychosocial factors related to the incidence of cancer." *International Journal of Psychiatry in Medicine,* 1978, 9:159–177.

Seligman, M.E.P. *Helplessness in depression, development, and death.* San Francisco: Freeman, 1975.

Selye, H. "A syndrome produced by diverse nocuous agents." *Na-*

ture, 1936, 138:32.

_____. "The general adaptation syndrome and the diseases of adaptation." *Journal of Clinical Endocrinology*, 1946, 6:117–230.

_____. *Stress: the physiology and pathology of exposure to systemic stress.* Montreal: Acta, Inc., 1950.

_____. *The story of the adaptation syndrome.* Montreal: Acta, Inc., 1952.

_____. *The stress of life.* New York: McGraw-Hill, 1956.

_____. *Hormones and resistance, Part 1.* New York: Springer, 1971.

_____. *Stress without distress.* Philadelphia: Lippincott, 1974.

_____. "Further thoughts on 'stress without distress.'" *Resident and Staff Physician*, April 1977:125–140.

Shapiro, D., Tursky, B., and Schwartz, G.E. "Differentiation of heart rate and blood pressures in man by operant conditioning." *Psychosomatic Medicine*, 1970, 32:417–423.

Shekelle, R.B. "Psychosocial factors and high blood pressure." *Cardiovascular Medicine*, 1979, 4:1249–1256.

Sholiton, L.J., Wohl, T.H., and Werk, E.E. "The correlation of adrenocortical function in patients with lung cancer." *Cancer*, 1963, 16:223–230.

Sigg, E.B. "The pharmacological approach to cardiac stress." In R.S. Eliot (ed.), *Stress and the heart.* New York: Futura, 1974.

Silver, B.V., and Blanchard, E.G. "Biofeedback and relaxation training in the treatment of psychophysiologic disorders: Or, are the machines really necessary?" *Journal of Behavioral Medicine*, 1978, 1:217–239.

Sklar, L.S., and Anisman, H. "Stress and cancer." *Psychological Bulletin*, 1981, 89:369–406.

Sternbach, R.A. *Pain patients, traits and treatment.* New York: Academic Press, 1974.

Suinn, R.M., Brock, L., and Edie, C. "Behavior therapy for Type A patients." *American Journal of Cardiology*, 1975, 36:269–270.

Swank, R.L. "Combat exhaustion." *Journal of Nervous and Mental Disease*, 1949, 109:475–508.

Tecce, J.J., Friedman, S.B., and Mason, J.W. "Anxiety, defensiveness, and 17-hydroxicorticosteroid excretion." *Journal of Nervous and*

Mental Disease, 1966, 141:549–554.

Tessler, R., Mechanic, D., and Dimond, M. "The effect of psychological distress on physician utilization: A prospective study." *Journal of Health and Social Behavior*, 1976, 17:353–364.

Theorell, T. "Selected illness and somatic factors in relation to two psychological stress indices: A prospective study on middle-aged construction workers." *Journal of Psychosomatic Research*, 1976, 20:7–20.

Theorell, T., Lind, E., Froberg, J., Karlsson, C.G., and Levi, L. "A longitudinal study of 21 subjects with coronary heart disease: Life changes, catecholamine excretion, and related biochemical reactions." *Psychosomatic Medicine*, 1972, 34:505–516.

Theorell, T., and Rahe, R.H. "Psychosocial factors and myocardial infarction: I—An inpatient study in Sweden." *Journal of Psychosomatic Research*, 1971, 15:25–31.

Thurlow, H.J. "Illness in relation to life situations and sick-role tendency." *Journal of Psychosomatic Research*, 1971, 15:73–88.

Tsuda, A., and Hirai, H. "Effects of the amount of required coping response tasks on gastrointestinal lesions in rats." *Japanese Psychological Research*, 1975, 17:119–132.

Turner, C.D. *General endocrinology*. 3rd ed. Philadelphia: Saunders, 1960.

Uhlenhuth, E.H., and Paykel, E.S. "Symptom configuration and life events." *Archives of General Psychiatry*, 1973A, 28:744–748.

_____. "Symptom intensity and life events." *Archives of General Psychiatry*, 1973B, 28:473–477.

Ursin, H., Baade, E., and Levine, S. *Psychobiology of stress—A study of coping men*. New York: Academic Press, 1978.

Venning, E.H., Dyrenfurth, I., and Beck, J.C. "Effect of anxiety upon aldosterone excretion in man." *Journal of Clinical Endocrinology*, 1957, 17:1005–1008.

Volicer, B. "Hospital stress and patient reports of pain and physical status." *Journal of Human Stress*, 1978, 4:28–37.

Volicer, B.J., Isenberg, M.A., and Burns, M.W. "Medical-surgical differences in hospital stress factors." *Journal of Human Stress*, 1977, 3:3–13.

Wadeson, R.W., Mason, J.W., Hamburg, D.A., and Handlon, J.H. "Plasma and urinary 17-OHCS responses to motion pictures." *Archives of General Psychiatry*, 1963, 9:146–156.

Weiner, H. *Psychobiology and human disease.* New York: Elsevier, 1977.

Weiss, J.M. "Somatic effects of predictable and unpredictable shock." *Psychosomatic Medicine*, 1970, 32:397–408.

———. "Psychological factors in stress and disease." *Scientific American*, 1972, 226:104–113.

Wershow, H.J., and Reinhart, G. "Life change and hospitalization – A heretical view." *Journal of Psychosomatic Research*, 1974, 18:393–401.

Westlund, K., and Nicolaysen, R. "Ten year mortality and morbidity related to serum cholesterol." *Scandinavian Journal of Clinical and Laboratory Investigation*, 1972, 30 (suppl. 127):1–24.

White, K., Williams, T.F., and Greenberg, B.G. "The ecology of medical care." *New England Journal of Medicine*, 1961, 265:885–892.

Wildman, R.C. "Life change with college grades as a role-performance variable." *Social Psychology*, 1978, 41:34–36.

Wildman, R.C., and Johnson, D.R. "Life change and Langner's 22-item mental health index: A study and partial replication." *Journal of Health and Social Behavior*, 1977, 18:179–188.

Williams, R.B. "Headache." In R.B. Williams and W.D. Gentry (eds.), *Behavioral approaches to medical treatment.* Cambridge, Massachusetts: Ballinger Publishing Company, 1977.

Wolf, S., and Goodell, H. *Stress and disease.* Springfield, Illinois: Charles C. Thomas, 1968.

Wolff, C.T., Friedman, S.B., Hofer, M.A., and Mason, J.W. "Relationship between psychological defenses and mean urinary 17-hydroxy-corticosteroid excretion rates: I – A predictive study of parents of fatally ill children." *Psychosomatic Medicine*, 1964, 26:576–591.

Wolff, C.T., Hofer, M.A., and Mason, J.W. "Relationship between psychological defenses and mean urinary 17-hydroxycorticosteroid excretion rates: II. – Methodological and theoretical considerations." *Psychosomatic Medicine*, 1964, 26:592–609.

Wooley, S.C., Blackwell, B., and Winget, C. "A learning theory model of chronic illness and behavior: Theory, treatment, and research." *Psychosomatic Medicine,* 1978, 40:379–401.

Wyatt, G.E. "A comparison of the scaling of Afro-Americans' life-change events." *Journal of Human Stress,* 1977, 3:13–21.

INDEX